**I have suffered from
bronchitis and respiratory problems for over ten
years. . . . As the bronchial condition worsened, I
was diagnosed as having asthma. . . .** It was the
week before Christmas when Dr. Koyfman began
treating me. After just a few treatments of colonics I
began to breathe better and feel stronger. . . .
—*J.M.*

**I had a chronic cough,
wheezing and shortness of breath** for one and one-
half years. . . . My chiropractor referred me to Dr.
Koyfman, and that referral changed my life. . . . I had
my first colonic and within three days the
coughing/wheezing was completely gone. . . .
—*D.C.*

**Our grandson was having
great difficulty breathing, and was supposed to
have sinus surgery.** Instead, we brought him to Dr.
Koyfman who worked with him for a little over two
months. Now our grandson is breathing normally
and is healthy. . . .
—*Family M.*

**Find the completion of
these testimonials in the chapter near the end of
the book entitled, "Testimonials."**

Healing through Cleansing

Book 1: Main Cleansing Channels

Colon

Kidneys

Lungs

Skin . . .

by Dr. Yakov Koyfman, N.D.

Practical Guide to a Healthy Lifestyle

Dedication

This little book is dedicated to the idea

That cleansing one's body of the toxins we take in
(from our food, water and air)
is an essential pathway to optimum health,

That natural techniques
which are gentle and powerfully effective
can and do remove the majority of these toxins,
and

That properly practicing
simple everyday cleansing procedures
is an important element
in one's overall detoxification program.

This book is one in a four-part series entitled:

Healing through Cleansing.

Book 1 is about the cleansing of the main excretory organs, the colon, kidneys, lungs and skin.

Book 2 tells how to cleanse the organs located in the head and neck region, the brain, thyroid gland, eyes, salivary glands, ears, nose and sinuses, throat, tongue, teeth and gums.

Book 3 deals with cleansing the abdominal organs, the stomach, small intestine, liver, blood vessels and blood, lymph, sexual organs, joints and spine.

Book 4 presents the main principles of a healthy diet with simple recipes for preparing living food dishes and safe cooking techniques which help to prepare freshly cooked foods without losing vital nutrients. Includes a weight loss program.

Each of these books contain testimonials both in the beginning and at the end of the book.

Preface

This book is published not as a substitute for, but rather as a supplement to, the care of your professional healthcare provider. More specifically, **the procedures described in this book are designed to support the body's immune system through cleansing specific internal organs and systems down to the cellular level.** In this way the body can be freed from the toxins it has picked up over the years, and its natural healing capacity strengthened. The information and techniques in this book are preventative in nature for the improvement of human health.

The information and the techniques described in this book are *not* designed to provide medical consultation or advice, diagnosis, prognosis, treatment procedures or prescription of remedies for any ailment or condition as those terms might be defined or construed by any federal, state or local law, rule, regulation or ordinance. Specifically, this book is not intended to engage in anything that legally would constitute the practice of medicine. The author of this book does not claim to treat any disease or provide any cure.

Instead, the information in this book is designed to create a better understanding of how the human body is capable of taking in and storing various chemicals, waste products and unwanted biologic organisms that are detrimental to human health. Further, this book is designed to discuss the impact these have on the human body, and how their partial or complete removal is beneficial to your health. Additionally, by increasing your awareness of these processes, this book hopes to create a greater self-awareness of personal health.

Because each person is unique, the author encourages each reader to pursue a daily self-care program tailored to his or her particular situation, based on that person's own best evaluation of the circumstances and in consultation with his or her professional healthcare provider.

Contents

Awaken! It is not Too Late... Yet

Two processes of destruction and rehabilitation lead the fight in the human body from the moment of birth and to the end of the life. When we are young, the rehabilitation process is dominating where as process of destruction is still weak and not as significant. However, when we reach approximately thirty years of age (or even sooner) the destruction process grows stronger making the rehabilitation process weaker.

So what exactly is being destructed in the human body?

The cells of the body become clogged and overfilled with toxicity, loose their elasticity and begin to age. Skin and tissue stretch and hang. Joint glands clog-up and produce less lubrication causing joint bones to rub against each other. Gradually joints rub off and coverup with salt crystals and uric acid. Polluted large intestine (colon) contaminates blood, blood vessels and lymph - slowing down circulation. The heart exhausts by trying to overcome the pressure in the colon and by pushing the blood through clogged-up vessels, and finally wears off. The energy drops drastically. Glands of internal secretion also become clogged. Lowers production and secretion of vital hormones. Slowly, but surely all organs and systems become congested and polluted, which significantly lowers their functioning. The body accumulates and produces more and more toxicity, and less nutrients to feed the immune system. The protection system weakens. Unfriendly bacteria, infection and other parasites meet less and less resistance from the immune system and reproduce easily. These creatures eat our nutrients, organs and muscles. They eat us alive! The body's resistance to destruction lowers rapidly and our unthoughtful actions speed up the process even more. The border line becomes closer and closer.

So how can you slow down that persistent stream of time?

In my books Healing Through Cleansing volumes 1-4, find answers on how to rid of many illnesses and stay healthy and young until a 100 and beyond.

xvi

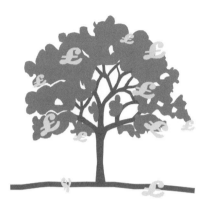

Introduction

In many ways our health depends on our lifestyle. Sometimes people who live an unhealthy lifestyle don't even know it because they don't understand what is a healthy lifestyle and what is an unhealthy lifestyle. Let's briefly describe these two ways of living.

An Unhealthy Lifestyle

An unhealthy lifestyle happens when you do not pay attention to your body and your health. People who live an unhealthy lifestyle assign either no time, or too little time, to improving their health. In addition, their diet and their lack of activity tends not toward improving health but toward destroying it. An unhealthy lifestyle pollutes and weakens the

1

whole system through the toxins it produces. Pollution to the system comes from poor diet, inactivity, poor blood and lymph circulation, lack of water and fresh air, wrong daily schedule, stresses and negative thinking, and also from the environment. Tiredness—being not just tired, but overtired, continuing to work or to work out when you feel tired, lack of rest and relaxation, and lack of sleep—is also related to an unhealthy lifestyle and increased pollution in the system.

A Healthy Lifestyle

A healthy lifestyle is the result of *the mind* having the knowledge it needs for good health, and *the will* having the wisdom and strength to implement that knowledge.

A healthy lifestyle is thinking, speaking, and acting in every way that leads to a **long life *and* high quality of living** without sacrificing any of the things in life that are truly enjoyable, profitable or natural.

A healthy lifestyle is **victory in living** not only for the physical body, but for the mind, the soul, and the spirit. As the body becomes healthier, so the mind thinks better and the soul and spirit become clearer.

A healthy lifestyle is **leaving behind the "pack mentality"** that is tragically symbolized by the lemmings that mythically race *en masse* over the proverbial cliff. It is not buying into *any* way of living that shortens your life or decreases the quality of living. It is not buying or using a product (or service) that is claimed to be good, but in reality is not. It is not allowing someone to treat your body with disrespect simply because he or she needs you to buy his or her product or service.

A healthy lifestyle is a **science** wherein the healing wisdom of the ages and the advantages of state-of-the-art medical science are blended together by both the experienced health professional and the informed patient.

A healthy lifestyle is an **art form** in which, once you have achieved your health goals through natural means, you walk through life exuding good health and leading others along the same victorious path.

A healthy lifestyle includes **cleansing your body** from toxins on all levels while faithfully maintaining that cleansing by following a rational diet.

Finally, a healthy lifestyle includes learning the necessary information about **proper exercise**, developing an exercise program tailored just for you, making time for that exercise program, and then actually doing the exercises on schedule.

People who live a healthy lifestyle constantly take care not just to cleanse the external body, but also to cleanse the internal organs. All of our organs and systems down to the cellular level require regular cleansing. Nature programs our bodies for this necessary maintenance to work automatically, but for many reasons our bodies become weak and cannot do this completely by themselves. They need help.

You—the individual in control of your body—are the first and most important element in achieving the optimum health possible for your body. Once you have decided to pursue this critical goal, you will need **reliable information**.

Our Center can recommend the following books to help guide you down the path of optimum health.

1. How to help clean your organs with professional help is described in my books: *Deep Internal Body Cleansing,* and *Eight Steps to Perfect Health.*
2. How to help your own system through self-help methods is described in my books, *Healing through Cleansing, Books 1-4,* and *Unique Method of Colon Rejuvenation.*

Where Do Health Problems Come from?

The answer to this question deserves a book in and of itself since the number of different chemical and biological toxins that cause so many of our diseases are as limitless as our ability to manufacture them. So instead of filling up page after page with the various harmful elements that are found in our food, water and air; it might be more interesting to examine this question in a context to which many in this country can relate.

A Day in the Life of an Average American

As diverse as Americans can be, there are some things that are basically the same for most adult Americans that go to work to earn a living outside of the home. A generic overview of a typical "day in the life" of an average American goes something like this:

1. Awakening to the blare of an alarm clock,
2. Plodding to the coffee pot in the kitchen to get that first cup of "go juice,"
3. Taking a shower, etc to help the coffee wake them up,
4. Eating a pre-manufactured breakfast at home,
5. Getting dressed while listening to the news about some tragedy somewhere,
6. Or reading the same negative news while having another

cup of coffee,

7. Driving to work through exhaust-flavored air while jostling with too many other weary souls, some of whom have divided their attention between driving and a cell phone,

8. Competing for a parking place,

9. Stopping for a fast food breakfast if they did not eat at home,

10. Working a job that, for most Americans, is not their true calling,

11. More coffee and maybe a cigarette,

12. Snacking from a machine or from some sugary goody that someone brought in,

13. Lunch: composed of non-organic foods grown on an industrial-type farm, shipped in from another state, and which have exceeded at least half of their shelf life while waiting to be nuked in a microwave that needs a tune-up,

14. More work that again does not satisfy their calling and true desire and in a work environment with some *really different* personalities,

15. More coffee and maybe a cigarette,

16. More sugary snacks with too much fat and processed flour,

17. Commute home in the company of numerous other speeding vehicles being driven by complete strangers who are as frazzled as you are, and who are listening to the same news about some unfortunate incident toward which you can only feel helpless,

18. Supper in a restaurant with more strangers, or eating more artificial foods at home alone   or with only some of the family present. The rest of the family is either caught in traffic or doing their own thing,

19. Watching contemporary television programming that is

as much junk food for the mind as the junk food you
put in your stomach earlier that day,

20. Alcohol,
21. Answering telemarketing telephone calls, evaluating
junk mail, and deleting junk emails,
22. Late night snacking on food that was sold to please
your tongue, not your nutritional needs,
23. Going to sleep in a house whose air has been bottled up
all day behind closed windows and doors,

What Is the Effect of All This on the Body?

The effects of such a lifestyle are both diverse and negative,
not many splendored. Impacts are measured physically,
emotionally, mentally and spiritually. Let's take a look at how
the body is affected by this barrage.

The Lungs

The sick air in your house and office, the exhaust-
contaminated air that your car's heater and AC pump into your
face during your two daily commutes, and the air in the various
businesses you visit come packaged with all kinds of invisible
airborne surprises. For example: carpet fibers, pet fur, dust,
dust mites, freon, vehicle exhaust which contains lead,
chemicals from hair sprays, and insect sprays, etc. These enter
the body unnoticed by the conscious mind, but not so
unnoticed by your body chemistry. While you are sleeping
your body and your heating/cooling system give off carbon
monoxide and carbon dioxide. Then there is the imperceptible

oxygen deficit from poor air exchange that leads to a slow poisoning of the cells. Centuries ago, most of these contaminants did not exist. But today they do, and we must be aware of them and their effect upon us. We must also take thoughtful, intelligent action to keep from having the problems that come with these toxins.

The Stomach, Small Intestine and Large Intestine

The typical American diet too often consists largely of dairy products that have been overly processed, meat, chips, sweets, fats, refined grain, canned food, and beverages (coffee, cola, ice water, beer, etc.). These products contain artificial hormones, antibiotics, food colorings, and other preservatives. As a result of these diet, fermentation starts inside the digestive system and good bacteria is destroyed. This in turn interferes with proper digestion, and causes a lot of gas and toxins to be formed, which then poisons the blood.

Muscles, Joints and Ligaments

From driving a car to driving a desk chair to piloting a remote control, the typical American does not get enough exercise. Back when this was an agricultural nation, such was not a problem, but all of those wonderful conveniences come with a price tag. These organs do not get enough movement, enough circulation, enough oxygen, or enough nutrition to stimulate them to optimal physical condition. However, they do get a large portion of the toxins we take into our bodies, which settle down in cells and intracellular spaces. These toxins not only poison these organs, but lead to pain.

The Nervous System

All that running around in traffic, the perception that you need to do more both faster and better, work-related stress, the constant (absolutely unrelenting) drive for more possessions and money, negative news reports and violent movies all add up. As a result we experience nervousness, fear, anger, disappointment, aggression, depression and other negative emotions which have a bad effect on our minds, spirits and energy fields. This situation in turn negatively affects us physically. And since nothing in our lives happens in a vacuum, we either repress these emotions or blast them out at others, which creates a whole new level of stress. Let's face it, very few people know how to discharge bad emotions safely the way excess electricity can be discharged into the ground.

The Liver

The liver is a filter and our primary cancer-fighting organ. As such, the river of bad chemicals that gets into the blood stream from all of the toxins we take in have to go here for proper treatment. In a sense, the liver takes the worst we have to offer, and sometimes gets so overwhelmed it stores toxic waste rather than sending it on to be eliminated. As a result of its function being impaired, digestion is weakened, toxins get in the blood poisoning it, liver stones are formed and the immune system is weakened. This lays the foundation for whatever disease is prevalent in your family.

The Kidneys

These twin filters are another organ that can be damaged by the unnatural chemicals that enter our bodies. If you want a prescription for how to damage these two all you need to do is consume large amounts of alcohol or other bad beverages, combined with too much salt, meat artificial chemicals. This will clog the kidneys, resulting in the formation of kidney sand, kidney stones, excess of protein in the urine, water retention in the body, and even an overload of the heart.

Other organs, tissues and fluids are also affected in bad ways. In fact, toxins hurt the body down to the cellular level. The only reason that you do not notice this poisoning is that it takes place little by little.

So How Do People Feel the Next Day?

After surviving the life style described above, a lot of people are not enjoying life at peak efficiency. In fact, getting up in the morning is a major effort. With toxin-encumbered organs and sluggish blood flowing through narrowed veins, an energy crisis of the most personal type is the order of the day. Frequently, such a person wakes up with sinus problems that clog the nasal passages, sore eyes and a white coating on the tongue. It is no surprise that they have a bad taste in their mouths, and are sometimes hoarse. At night, the manmade chemicals (which have created a chemical imbalance) and the emotion of the day can combine to produce nightmares. Additionally, the body can alternate between being very hot or very cold during sleep. When morning arrives, stimulants such as coffee or other forms of caffeine/nicotine are needed to get passed the somnambulist stage.

So What Are the Alternatives?

The first thing to do is to get a thorough understanding of :
1. How toxins get into your body.
2. How toxins affect your health.
3. How to remove toxins effectively.
4. How to maintain a toxin-free body for maximum health.

Once you have done this, you can wake up with a smile, with your sinus' wide open for easy breathing and lots of oxygen. This will help your eyes to shine and your tongue to be clean and healthy pink. A night's rest will be exactly that, so that you wake up refreshed and energized. You will welcome each day and actually enjoy waking up in the morning. You will feel more creative, and have a firm confidence that your physical and mental health is normal.

If enjoying life at this level is something you genuinely want, then you will find a wealth of useful, practical information in this book. If you want the highest quality physical health you can obtain for yourself, then understanding and implementing the knowledge and techniques in this book will be of great benefit. Of course, you will have to invest some effort. This is not done while surfing television or the net. Nor is it accomplished with a mouthful of potato chips. One has to engage the most powerful healer of all— the mind—and to steer oneself up the road to maximum health. And one must "marry" the heart to the mind to bring the desires of the heart in harmony with the strength of the mind. With these two operating together, and armed with the knowledge and procedures in this book, you can rid yourself of the toxins that damage your personal health and become "clear."

Understand that the information in this book was not pulled

out of thin air. It is based on thousands and thousands of years of alternative medicine, yoga, and other natural healing disciplines. It is also based on a quarter century of personal research in both Europe and America. So this is not just theorizing or simply book learning. Everything in this book is part of my personal everyday practice, and has been successfully utilized by numerous clients over the last 25+ years.

Remember: Whatever goals you have in life—spiritual, career, athletic, romantic, etc.—can be better accomplished from optimum health.

To learn more about unique cleansing procedures done in our center, please visit our website at
www.koyfmancenter.com

Good News!

For many years I suffered from many health conditions, including breathing difficulties, skin eruptions, muscular twitching, joint and back pain, and others. I went from one medical doctor to another trying to find answers and help; only to hear bad news. Nevertheless, I declined all of their prescriptions and decided to investigate the alternatives for myself. Then I was referred to Dr. Koyfman. Finally, I began to hear some good news. He explained the problem of toxins and parasites and told me that he believed he could help me. Good news indeed! I began to follow his recommendations which included cleansings of the colon, digestive system, small intestine, liver and lymphatic system. The results were both dramatic and progressive. The symptoms (all of them) began to diminish steadily until by the time I completed the recommended procedures, they were either completely gone or nearly gone. I am deeply grateful to Dr. and Mrs. Koyfman, their family and staff for their courteous, kind, and professional care given to me during this time. Because of them I am feeling better than I have felt in a very long time and hope to continue my cleansings for as long as I live.

-Hank Taylor-

My Seven-Year-Old Son is Grateful

He's been suffering from constipation for a long time. His digestion was not good at all. He began feeling tired and did not perform well in school. During his first cleansing procedure an unbelievable amount of waste came out. Dr. Koyfman modified his diet and daily regiment. Now my boy has a b.m. on his own every day. It is not painful anymore. He is playing sports and his concentration is much better. **-A Happy mom.**

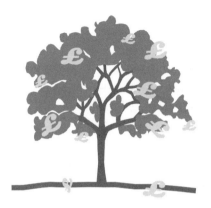

The Pathway to Optimal Health

Do You Really Need to See a Doctor?

The sheer force of medical research, both alternative medicine and traditional medicine, has been steadily driving our understanding of healing towards the importance of internal body cleansing. Vast amounts of money, time and talent are spent each year on understanding how the body works. Since the human body is, in one sense, a very intricate chemical factory, understanding how that chemistry is balanced is the leading answer to most health and healing questions.

Because of this, the media is full of information supporting the simple idea that "toxins in the body poison the body." The

13

idea is so basic that it is inescapable. Who could anyone possibly deny that if you put a low grade poison (toxins) into your body that your health would degrade? And who could possibly deny that if you remove a low grade poison (toxins) that your health would improve? Even traditional doctors are coming around to this unavoidable concept.

On the other hand, the pharmaceutical companies, who make their money by putting chemicals into you, are the only ones opposed to the basic concept of removing manmade chemicals from the body for the purpose of healing. They rightly realize that internal body cleansing will erode their bottom line. After all, the legitimate need for pharmaceuticals is relatively small, and useful really only for emergency situations. Once the majority of people realize this, drug sales will shrink. They know that their market ($) is dependant on winning in the marketplace of ideas, so the blitzkrieg of advertising continues.

Please keep in mind that pharmaceuticals (drugs) are generally not designed, marketed, advertised or sold to change the basic lifestyle or mind set of anyone. They are really meant to treat symptoms or create a new balance in which symptoms improve, at least temporarily. Granted some drugs can cure certain problems. Some drugs literally kill a disease. But by and large pharmaceuticals are really a balancing act that changes an already out-of-balance personal chemistry. Just because the body's chemistry has become unbalanced in one direction is no reason to try to fix it by over-correcting it in the other extreme. The best idea is to return the body's chemistry to its original, natural balance in which no artificial chemicals are present. Keep the scales level.

So why visit the doctor to get drugs? Instead of trying to tip the scales with a new weight (drugs), return your health to natural chemistry. Because once you start down this path, you may well be causing "the bad health dominoes" to begin falling. And once they do most people end up trying to compensate with more of the same.

The reason to visit any medical professional's office is not discuss the problems, but to find the cause of the problems. If the problem is a broken bone, surely traditional medicine is a good thing. Indeed, traditional medicine is quite capable of providing some very important and beneficial services, such as in the emergency room. But when it comes to problems caused by the toxicity of the body, they have yet to stop treating the problem with the problem: more drugs.

Most people in this country understand and support the idea of a "drug-free America." In this context the discussion is about illegal drugs. While I am not putting the products of the pharmaceutical industry in the same basket as illegal drugs, I am trying to get you to think of the basic principles behind them both. Illegal drugs are bad (very bad) because of the negative impact they have on the mind, body, soul and society. If a legal drug (over the counter or prescription) merely relieves symptoms and does not cure **when there is** a real way of preventing or quashing an illness then the legal drug and its advertising are getting in the way of real healing. And this is not to mention the side effects that come packaged with some legal drugs. Drugs like thalidomide and others that cause birth defects or damaged organs, etc. Cleansing the body of toxins never has this problem because it never introduces an artificial chemical. It only restores natural chemical balance. Nature knows what it is doing. Stick with the basic plan laid out by nature, and do not mess with the chemistry.

15

What is Toxicity?

Toxins are really any chemical (organic or inorganic) that degrades the health of the body regardless of the length of time it takes to operate. This is in contrast to vitamins, minerals, etc that increase the health of the body.

It is a this point that we run head-on into a little problem. We have to eat food and drink water to stay alive. But no food is a perfect food, and our digestive systems are not perfect in their jobs. Because of this even the most organic vegetarian diet will create toxins in the body. This is because as food is not pure vitamins, minerals, etc. Food contains a wide variety of substances that the body can not use and will not digest. This part of our food has to be removed by the excretory organs: the intestinal tract, the urinary tract, the sweat glands and the lungs.

Here's where the problems begin even for those on "the perfect diet." Solid waste matter passing through the colon (feces) are somewhat sticky, and will adhere to the walls of the large intestine. This waste becomes stuck to the colon walls for years and years. Over the decades it gets thicker and thicker. As this material—which the body has already rejected—rots in place, harmful chemicals are given off. These bad chemicals pass through the colon walls and enter the blood stream. They are then carried throughout the body, and are stored in various organs and tissues where they interfere with the functioning of that organ. This is where we get toxicity-derived illnesses and diseases. It is the presence of these unwanted chemicals that is the root of the problem experienced as symptoms. Additional chemicals (pharmaceuticals) are not the answer. Removing these bad chemicals is the answer.

In the case of the typical American diet composed of coffee, sugar, fats, processed foods, food preservatives, food additives, alcohol, et cetera ad infinitum, the chemical situation becomes much worse. These unnatural chemicals become stuck to the colon walls with all the rest of the indigestible food and are eventually returned to the blood stream. They too are stored throughout the body and weaken health thereby. After all, the various organs, tissues and cells never asked for these unknown chemicals. They were never programmed for these chemicals and have no idea how to deal with them.

Now the immune system tries to deal with these foreign chemicals. Since most Americans have a habit of stuffing themselves with large quantities of processed foods full of these unhappy compounds, the immune system has a mighty chore for itself. Over the years, the immune system can become overwhelmed. With the immune system tied down in fighting this powerful toxic foe, colds and flu have a much stronger chance of running at fever pitch in your weakened body. Even worse, genetically inherited diseases have an increased opportunity to develop and grow with the immune system in a weakened state.

Individuals who have had colonics (discussed below) have proven beyond all doubt that this waste does get stuck to the colon walls, and has already rotted to a blackened (anaerobic) waste that is nothing like what would otherwise leave the body. They know that it is more than simply excess weight that is measured every time they got on the scales. They know that this waste creates an oxygen-starved environment in the colon; one in which good bacteria used for proper digestion can not live. They know they want that poison out of the body.

As soon as this waste is removed from the colon by simply washing it out with a colonic, the immune system can begin to play catch-up on the toxins stored throughout the body. If one elects to do other cleanses for specific organs to remove those wastes, then the immune system will have a very light load and can concentrate its energy on colds, flu, and genetically inherited diseases. After all, the human body is nature's greatest doctor, and if we let it do what it knows how to do, it will do it with great skill. In time, this great internal healer will re-establish all systems to normal, assuming some genetic defect or outside agency does not interfere.

It goes without saying that you should also have a proper diet, and do exercises appropriate for your personal situation. Add to this mental and emotional health techniques and you will create a delightful balance for the entirety of your being that few around you will have. This total balance will benefit every aspect of your life.

Types of Cleansing Procedures

Cleansing the body of toxins can be grouped into two separate categories:
1. **Daily cleansing procedures** which anyone can do by themselves, and
2. **Deep internal body cleansing** performed by health professionals.

Let's break these two categories up just a little bit further into five levels.

Level I   Cleansing the outside of our bodies by doing things such as showering/bathing, brushing our teeth, washing our hair, cleaning under our fingernails, etc. (It has been reported that one of the nastiest places on the human body is under the fingernails.) Don't underestimate the importance of these simple cleanses. They

18

should be ingrained as daily habits.

Now ask yourself this question: Is there a way to go deep into the body without traumatizing it (i.e. without using a scalpel) to get rid of accumulated wastes? The answer is: If there is a way forward, then there has to be a way back. Or in other words, **if the toxins have a path in, they have a path out. All we have to do is open the door and urge them out.**

Level II	Cleansing internal organs which can be easily reached, such as the colon, sinuses, and ears.
Level III	Cleansing the organs which are not easily reached. These organs can be cleansed through the channels of other organs which are connected to them. This would include the liver, the kidneys, the stomach, the small intestine, the lymph system, the pancreas, etc. For example: the liver excretes wastes into the small intestine which in turn empties into the colon, which has an exit to the outside. Therefore, liver can be cleansed through the small and large intestine.
Level IV	Cellular cleansing which is achieved with the help of fasting, and supported by the cleansing action of the colon, kidneys, skin, lungs, etc.
Level V	The cleansing the mind and body from harmful emotional wastes. These include such negative emotions as: anger, jealousy, fear, envy, hate, helplessness, and sadness. These emotions generate negative energies inside the body that

create large emotional blocks, and non-stop stress on all or part of muscles and organs. This stress slowly sucks the energy out of the body, and creates more blocks. To overcome this stress, the mind and body expend a lot of time and energy. During this process physical wastes are generated, sometimes on a large scale.

Cleansing the mind and body of emotional wastes can be achieved through:
1. Cleansing and massaging internal organs such as the: stomach, small intestine, liver, diaphragm, heart. These organs are the sites of the greatest waste accumulation.
2. Relaxing massages (Emotional wastes are also found in muscles.)
3. Respiratory exercises such as yoga and long walks outside.
4. Relaxation, meditation and prayer.
5. Consciously controlling emotions.
6. The decreased affinity for material possessions.
7. Forgiveness of others and yourself. (Very powerful)
8. Self-assurance in the positive outcome of the cleansing program.

Daily cleansing consists of the things our bodies automatically do whenever we get ill, and the common hygienic procedures we are already doing (Level I above), but with a conscious intent to make these everyday habits a vital part of our health maintenance program. By properly performing such procedures as showering, bathing, teeth brushing, etc., we are engaged in assisting all of the excretory organs and the channels of waste removal. These organs and channels are:

1. **Colon** - a universal channel of excretion of solid, liquid, mucous and gaseous toxins.
2. **Kidneys** - excretion of mainly liquid, dissolved toxins, mucous and even solids such as sand, salts, and sometimes kidney stones.
3. **Skin** - for the most part this is the channel of removal of liquid, dissolved toxins.
4. **Lungs** - the channel of excretion of gaseous toxins, which are passed through bronchial and nasal passages. Nasal passages are also channels for excreting mucous toxins from the sinuses.

We will name these four organs the main excretory organs. **It is important to concentrate on the main excretory organs because they are the means by which the largest amount of toxins can be removed from the body, and because they are your connection to the rest of the body for removing toxins from other organs, glands, cells, and tissues.**

To summarize, deep cleansing on all levels is achieved through freeing it from physical and emotional wastes. A major part of this kind of cleansing is done in clinical conditions under professional supervision, however there are still a great deal one can do at home.

Important Principle of Cleansing

It is vital to realize that **by cleansing one organ you partly cleanse and stimulate other adjacent organs.** *For example: by cleansing the lungs we also cleanse the sinuses, bronchial and nasal passages. By cleansing our skin we are also helping kidneys, lungs, etc.*
When you master the techniques of helping the main

excretory organs, try to incorporate the rest of the cleansing procedures. Regular help to all excretory channels of the body plays a major role in maintenance of good health.

How Do You Find Time for Daily Cleansing Procedures?

The easiest part of doing daily cleansing procedures is that they take almost no extra time. This is because we are just upgrading what we are already doing by improving our attitude and technique. Once we understand that these seemingly run-of-the-mill hygienic "chores" can have deeper health benefits if seen as part of the overall health picture, we then employ this knowledge to greater effect.

For example:

1. During every visit to the bathroom we also spend time cleansing the colon by including one or more simple colon exercises to increase the amount of waste expelled.
2. The time that we use to take a shower includes cleansing blood vessels as the hot shower water causes toxins to leave through the skin.
3. Brushing our teeth removes tiny food particles from the mouth that otherwise rot.
4. When we take a walk outside we spend are also cleansing our lungs and calming our emotions.

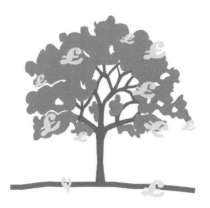

The Role of the Mind

How Can Cleansing Procedures Be Improved by Conscious Thought?

Even if you do not focus your mind completely on the cleansing procedure while you are doing it, you will still get some benefit from it. However, by engaging your mind deliberately on what you are doing and why you are doing it you will greatly increase its effect on your health. This is especially true if you make this focus a habit.

Psychological Power and Effects of Thought

To better understand how thought helps the body cleanse and heal itself, let's look more closely at what "thought" is, and how it interacts with the body. Thought is psychological energy. This energy is generated by and flows from all of the other types of energy created in the body: digestion, nervous, chemical, thermal, electrical, magnetic and spiritual. With the help of thought energy you can consciously and subconsciously control all of your physical, mental, emotional, moral and spiritual processes.

Since all of these processes directly and indirectly relate to physical health, your thought life is of critical importance to achieving and maintaining your bodily well-being. More than a few persons have learned to focus their thoughts so that the power of the mind stimulates the immune system and other systems of the body to direct their massive healing powers against specific illnesses. Even traditional doctors will not deny the power of the mind to heal when all of their techniques have failed. Again, the mind is the most powerful organ in the body. It is the one who makes the choices that determine so many aspects of our lives.

Negative Emotions and Toxicity

Often our thoughts are not under our conscious control. Instead, most people simply let their thoughts run loosely much like the caprices of the wind. One thought follows another in a random way without any defined goal. In our mind we argue with the boss, prove something to our relatives, friends or co-workers. A great deal of time our mental debates focus on situations which generate negative emotions: revenge, fear, jealousy, anger, etc. These kinds of thoughts bring with them their own kind of anxiety, which disturbs the natural harmony we could otherwise have. Without really meaning to we set ourselves up for stress and depression.

What Happens in Our Bodies at That Time?

Negative emotions created by our negative thoughts first disrupt the balance in the energy fields in our bodies. Then they create tension in corresponding internal organs. Blockages form in these organs resulting in a disruption in blood circulation, bile flow, digestion and energy circulation. Metabolic processes are also disrupted. Since nothing happens in a vacuum, these disturbances result in the creation of physical and emotional wastes that poison both mind and body. This leads to the inevitable conclusion that **the body gets poisoned not only from improper diet but also from improper thinking.**

How Can You Learn Not to Think?

One of the most effective and basic techniques for controlling one's thought life is to "give it a rest." To begin this process learn to ask yourself, *"What am I thinking about right now?"* If it turns out that you are thinking negatively, switch the direction of your thoughts. Or even better, give yourself a break from your thoughts. Tell yourself, "*I am not thinking about anything. I am monitoring my thoughts.*" And as soon as any thought starts to form, don't follow it, don't analyze it, don't stress over it, but try to let it go. Then wait for the next thought and once again let it go. After regular training you will notice that the "thoughtless" period is getting longer and longer. This will allow you to not think for 5-10 minutes; and help your mind, emotions, body and spirit to rest. After this kind of relaxation your mind will be clear and light.

"Gotta Change My Way of Thinking"

Once you have learned to clear your mind of stray thoughts you will want to learn to fill it with positive thoughts, particularly in the context of healing. To achieve this during cleansing procedures you should think, or even mentally repeat, positive statements which will help to paint the picture of what it is you are trying to achieve. In time, regular repetition of this process will help you to clearly visualize your goal.

For example: **Old Way of Thinking:** *"I am taking a shower."* **New Way of Thinking:** *"I am cleansing the pores of my skin, and improving my respiration through my skin.* **Old Way of Thinking:** *"I am going for a walk."* **New Way of Thinking:** *"I am cleansing my lungs from stagnant air, saturating my cells with oxygen, and cleansing and calming my mind."* The list is endless, especially when you begin to incorporate into your lifestyle these simple principles. A hidden benefit of this process is that you will naturally begin to focus on the little things in your life, and evaluate them for their health value. When you find a bad practice, you will ease it out of your life and yourself on towards greater health.

In the past, you were performing a cleansing procedure as a

chore not completely realizing what you were doing. Your uncontrolled thoughts were all over the place instead of being with you and focused beneficially on your actions. Now when performing a cleansing procedure you are supplementing your actions with positive mental images. In other words you understand (thought) what you are doing and you supplement it with your imagination (image). If you learn to combine your actions and your thoughts into a single process, your success will be much more effective.

Once again I'd like to emphasize the importance of positive thinking. It is especially relevant for those who are skeptical about these procedures. It is perfectly normal if you don't completely believe in this at first. Most importantly don't dismiss it without testing it out. Reread this chapter. Find more literature on this topic. Broaden your knowledge. Research this yourself. And best of all, field test it to prove it to yourself.

The Effect of Thought on the Hormonal System

All of us have had experiences that demonstrate that physical process can be started merely by certain thoughts. Take for example oversleeping on a work day. You open one sleepy eye and look at your clock only to realize that will be late for work. Instantly you are wide awake (immediate change in mental state.) Your heartbeat goes from slow to fast in the space of one beat. You jump out of bed, proving that your muscles can go from a state of rest to full capacity in the span of a thought. Once on your feet, your movements are at a speed more like you have been awake for an hour than fresh out of bed. Adrenaline has been dumped into your blood, and you are thinking and moving at full speed. Your breathing becomes deeper, digestion slows down, and your emotions (fear, anger, anxiety, etc.) are working just as energetically as your muscles.

If that example did not make the point, simply recall the last really bad near-miss you had in traffic with some other driver. Time itself becomes distorted as your mind focuses on the danger at hand. This has been reported by numerous police officers caught in gun fights with criminals. Some officers have reported being shot and not realized it because of the overwhelming emotions of the situation. The adrenaline and hormones blocked out everything but the threat. Tunnel vision set in.

Thought is a great power. A disciplined mind, trained to control its thoughts, can achieve nearly anything. Everything that has been accomplished by the human race in technical progress, medicine, arts and other areas started with a thought. It may have been driven by passion, but it was realized first.

The Value of Knowing the Therapeutic Effects of Cleansing Procedures

Understanding the health benefits of a given procedure, exercise or massage plays a very important role in achieving maximum results. Keeping these benefits in mind while you are undergoing a given procedure is even more powerful because the mind is able to enhance the positive effects of the procedure by directing the organ or system in harmony with it. This is done by the mental focus increasing the energy of a given organ, increasing blood flow and acting as a form of self-hypnosis.

This technique is simple. During the cleansing procedure, exercise or massage, concentrate your attention on the organ being cleansed and visualize its cleansing. Think about how this organ is becoming cleaner, improving in functioning, becomes stronger and more productive. The more you will think and imagine that your organs and cells are strong and healthy, the stronger is your body going to be as a whole. But your positive thoughts should be based on those positive actions that you do to improve your health. There is not much use for positive thoughts accompanied by harmful actions (overeating, not moving much, polluting the body with harmful beverages and food, etc). This book gives you a wide assortment of procedures, exercises and massages beneficial for your health. It is here, on this background, that positive thoughts, emotions and images will play a great role in strengthening your health.

God-given Birthright

I thank God for the awareness and guidance that led me to visit the Koyfman Center. With Dr. Koyfman's expertise and thorough attention and care of the staff/family, I eventually came to think of the center as the foundation of my physical health plan!

The people at the Koyfman Center supported and assisted me in cleansing the body all the way to the cellular level allowing me to rebuild and reprogram ALL systems, including emotional and mental. The body, the food, the addictions or craving no longer have any power! I now claim my God-given birthright of radiant health and beauty. I have learned to understand my body's language and have designed a maintenance program to support my systems in a manner that works beautifully for me. I am blessed to be feeling stronger and healthier each day.

Many Thanks and Blessings to the Koyfmans and Helen for the huge part they have played in my journey of HEALTH!

If you are reading this at the Koyfman Whole Body Cleansing, that tells me you are about to give yourself a great gift. I wish you blessings and health.

For information or support, feel free to e-mail me at:
fryrwellbeing@yahoo.com
Barbara Murray, Age 48
Tennessee

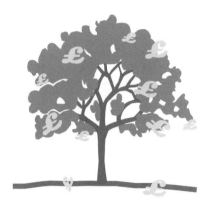

The Colon

How to Help the Large Intestine to Clean Itself

Structure and Function of the Large Intestine:

The large intestine is a pipe-like channel 5 to 6 feet in length. It starts in the bottom right of the abdominal cavity, goes up (ascending colon), then turns to the left and goes across the abdomen (transverse colon), goes down on the left (descending colon), makes a loop (sigmoid), becomes narrower and ends with an exit to the outside (anus), from which the fecal masses are excreted. In the bottom right part of the intestine a structure called the appendix is located.

The absorption of nutrients occurs in the small intestine.

Everything that is left over goes into the large intestine, and from there is expelled from the body. So the function of the large intestine is to remove the waste from the body. As a result of the consumption of refined food products, improper food combinations, overeating, stress, not enough water, etc. fecal masses in the colon become dehydrated. These dehydrated wastes stick to the sides of the intestine, creating a thick coating down its length. As a result of this, **the large intestine becomes the best place to store "trash" and the most polluted organ of the body. This trash rots in place releasing toxins that from thence spread throughout the entire body.**

Constipation

Most people have constipation in one form or another, to one degree or another. Often they do not even realize it because it is so mild that it is hidden to them. Unfortunately, **constipation is the beginning link in a chain of very dangerous diseases, the worst of which is cancer.**

When constipation is obvious a person may not go to the bathroom for 1 day to even 2 weeks. Their stools are hard and difficult to pass.

In the hidden form a person will likely go to the bathroom daily, even twice a day, but the excreted amount is very small in volume. Sometimes constipation changes into diarrhea, but both of these point to an imbalance inside their system. This imbalance can be in the micro flora or bacteria in the colon, the presence of parasites, or decay or putrefaction of wastes.

If a person eats three times a day, then he gets 21 meals in a week. If his large intestine is functioning only once a day (which many people consider normal), then this makes for 7 visits to the bathroom during a week. What about another 14 excretions? Remember, he ate 21 times but visited the bathroom only 7 times. Where did all of it go and why is there no balance?

Of course, the entire volume of food we eat is not excreted by the body. The nutrients in food are isolated, absorbed into the blood and delivered to our organs, cells and tissues. The fiber from vegetables, fruits, grains, products of metabolism and dead cells, etc are excreted in the form of feces.

So what happens to the fats, starches, and refined products which do not contain fiber? These sticky, glue-like substances are left on the walls of the intestine, settling there layer by layer, and clogging the passageway. Eventually, the colon can become blocked. Examples of this are found throughout American society, including famous people. Actor John Wayne died with 78 pounds of this fecal material in his colon, and Elvis Presley (who liked to eat *fried* peanut butter sandwiches) died straining on the toilet. You don't have to be famous to have these problems. All you have to do is eat bad food and neglect proper cleansing.

Improper food combinations and processed foods react poorly in the digestive tract causing foods there to become sticky like uncooked dough made from white flour. This stickiness causes the digesting food to move slowly, sometimes very slowly, through the small intestine and large intestine. If this material were moving at a healthy rate, nutrients would be removed, and the material the body normally rejects would be quickly escorted out. Unfortunately, this material has time in the colon to rot, causing nutrients to be degraded to the point of being inferior or unusable. A significant part of improper combinations (proteins and starches) are not absorbed, and settle on the walls of the large intestine. Gradually the walls of the large intestine become covered with old wastes. This builds a barrier between the colon walls (which are designed to remove nutrients) and the newly arriving foods that have the nutrients your body needs.

This has the unhappy result of (1) prohibiting the absorption of fresh nutrients, (2) allowing the absorption of old and decayed nutrients, and (3) physically resisting the normal contractions (peristalsis) of the colon. That's why in many people the intestine functions only after the arrival of new food, i.e. from the push from above and not from the muscle activity of the large intestine.

As the "plaque" on the walls of the intestine increases, the diameter of the *passageway* decreases. This restricts the normal flow of material through the colon and causes the large intestine to begin to lose its function. To fight constipation, many people use laxatives. This is not a good idea. Laxatives may seem to help, but only in the removal of food recently eaten. Although freed up from most of the recent material "in the pipeline," only the worst symptoms have been dealt with. The original problem has not changed. Obvious constipation returns, and an even larger dose of laxatives is consumed by the sufferer.

Laxatives are just another chemical added to your personal body chemistry. They are composed of artificial chemicals cooked up in an industrial laboratory. Laxatives irritate the colon walls, poison it slowly, and cause this long tubular muscle to spasm to get the results the person thinks he wants. This spasming of the colon causes it to flex and twist. This unnatural movement, over time, leads to changes in the normal shape of the colon such as enlargements and constrictions. The situation has only gotten worse.

Blocked Large Intestine and Parasites

Under these circumstances, the large intestine becomes an elongated storage bin of decomposing feces that release poisons into the bloodstream and create an oxygen-poor environment well-suited for harmful bacteria and parasites. Parasites are not known for having a discriminating palate. They will eat just about anything. This includes the rotting material in your colon, your own body tissues, and the fresh food you had at your last meal or snack. This creates a three-fold problem: (1) you are now competing for limited nutrients in your food with an ugly, unwelcome "squatter" who cares nothing for your health, (2) the little monster will eat the very tissues of your body setting in motion a wide range of new health problems, and (3) even if you fast it can feed off of the waste stuck to your colon. This means you can not starve it out.

Now the problem gets worse. Parasites excrete wastes themselves, which in turn poison your personal body chemistry. It is bad enough to have your own wastes stuck in your body releasing toxins into your blood stream, but to have a host of these nasty creatures in you dumping their wastes into your blood stream is an awful picture. And do not imagine that all parasites are microscopic, or so small that you can barely see them. Numerous books on parasites have reported persons in developed countries (including North America) having parasites as long as several feet. A 19 pound parasite was accidently discovered in one obese woman during surgery. Worms that long can put out a lot of poison.

If that was not bad enough, parasites will often lay eggs in their host. Now the hapless person is set up for a lifetime of parasitic invasion. (This is almost inconceivable for the average American who thinks parasites are only a problem in third world countries. But if you have ever had a pet or eaten in a restaurant you have had ample opportunity to be exposed.) No one wants to think of themselves as a "parasite hotel," but the sad truth is that the eggs laid in the walls of your colon hatch, and new generations of parasites spread throughout the entire body. Tiredness, weakness, colds, allergies, skin problems, gasses, some pains, depressions and tens of other conditions and serious diseases can be the result. And it all really starts with constipation that gave these foreign life forms a place to grow.

Another Unrecognized (Hidden) Reason for Constipation

Sometimes, the urge to go to the bathroom may come at a moment when you really can not get to the facilities. For example, you may be in a meeting or traveling in a car. In contrast you may get the signal when you are doing something you really like, but could make it to the bathroom if you so chose. Unfortunately this natural signal has come at "a bad time," so you decide to put it off because you don't want to interrupt whatever it is you are doing for such an "unimportant" event.

Lets examine what happens in the body when you use your will power to block this natural signal. When the process of digestion is completed, the body chooses to get rid of what it has deemed to be a foreign substance. The colon goes about making this happen by pushing the wastes to the exit. When these wastes get close to the exit (rectum) they stop because the exit is closed by a valve called the sphincter muscle. For this exit to open it takes both position and a certain amount of pressure from the wastes. When the large intestine is so full that its contents are pushing on its walls, it reacts by squeezing. The pressure of the wastes on the valve increases, and you feel the signal to go to the bathroom. If you ignore this signal, the large intestine becomes quiet for a while, and then repeats the squeezing in its attempt to eliminate wastes. This process of signaling and holding followed by more signaling and holding can be repeated several to many times depending on the person.

While your colon is waiting for permission to release, more wastes are being collected in the lower part of the large intestine. As wastes build up, the diameter of the colon increases and the pressure from this mass creates an uncomfortable heaviness in that area. When your colon realizes that its attempts to get rid of wastes and excess pressure are ignored, it stops squeezing because that only increases the pressure.

The large intestine is then forced to try to relieve the pressure in a different way. It starts to absorb water from the wastes. As the wastes become dehydrated, their volume decreases and the pressure inside the intestine goes down. However, there are side effects to this secondary solution. The dehydration of the wastes causes them to become hardened. Additionally, the water absorbed from the waste contains toxins, which instead of being ejected pass through the walls of the colon and enter the bloodstream. The circulatory system spreads these toxins to other organs, polluting and poisoning them.

When in a few hours, or even the next day, new food enters the intestine, it again increases the pressure on the walls, stimulating you to finally go to the bathroom. There you may notice symptoms of constipation. For example it is hard to eliminate waste especially when you first try. This is because the feces have become hardened by their loss of lubricating water, and it is therefore more difficult for them to slide down the colon walls. In addition, because of their increase in diameter they press more tightly against the walls of the colon, especially in the lower colon. This may require heavy pressure for their elimination sometimes creating internal or external hemorrhoids. If you often ignore the natural signal to eliminate, you can develop serious constipation with all of the bad consequences.

In conclusion I'd like to quote a great yoga master, thinker and doctor Swami Sevananda: **"If you are in doubt whether to go to the bathroom or not - go! If you are in doubt whether to eat or not - don't eat!"**

Physical and Chemical Effects of a Distended Large Intestine on Other Organs

In the case of a large intestine that has become coated with multiple layers of old wastes, both the diameter and the weight of the colon increase, creating new forms of harmful side effects. The now extended volume of the colon takes up two, three or more times as much space than it was ever designed to do. This decreases the "living space" of adjacent organs, pushing them aside and inhibiting their normal functioning by the unnatural pressure placed on these surrounding organs. For example, the excess volume of wastes and gases can push on the heart, making it work under abnormal conditions, causing it to wear out faster.

As if the change in volume were not enough of a problem, the weight of these accumulated wastes push down on the organs below them, compressing them. This particularly affects the urinary tract, and the blood flow in the sex organs, both male and female. Because of this a lot of men and women start experiencing problems with these organs, especially after age 40. This unnatural weight also has an unhappy effect on the organs above the colon by pulling them downward and stretching ligaments. Naturally these problems did not happen to us overnight, and require some time for their proper correction.

How Can You Determine the Condition of Your Large Intestine?

Eastern medicine has a simple, three-level method of determining the health of the large intestine. Locate the sigmoidal portion of your large intestine with your hand. Using **light pressure** only, press on this portion of your colon. If you experience pain, you have a serious problem. If you passed this test, press in the same location with **moderate pressure.** If you felt pain at this pressure level, the problem is not as serious. If you passed both of these two tests use **heavy pressure** on the sigmoid portion of your colon. If after a heavy pressure there is no pain the large intestine is in good condition.

Important Conclusion

To make sure that the large intestine is in good health you have to get it clean, and then keep it clean. If you had never had your large intestine properly cleansed before it is necessary to undergo a series of colon cleansings (colonics), and then maintain this cleanliness by doing regular colonics. But to be sure that the large intestine is in its best shape you have to take care of it daily.

The List of Daily Procedures

Some of the basic daily techniques for proper colon health include:

1. Eating correctly in order to supply the muscles of the large intestine with sufficient amounts of living enzymes, vitamins, minerals and plant fiber.
2. Drinking sufficient amounts of healthy liquids (according to your weight, level of physical activity, individual physique and the season of the year.)
3. Going to the bathroom as soon as you feel the need. The unnatural delay puts extra stress on the muscles of the intestine and makes them weaker.
4. Performing special **cleansing exercises** to strengthen the muscles of the large intestine and helping it to eliminate wastes completely.

Let's Briefly Describe the Concept of *Cleansing Exercises*

Remember: The body does a large percentage of its self-healing while you are asleep. This natural healing cycle naturally generates a lot of waste as the body gets rid of dead cells, etc.

When you wake up in the morning, the first thing you should do is to drink 2 - 3 glasses of water with lemon juice.

(This should be juice you have freshly squeezed from a lemon, not lemon juice from a bottle or can.)

Right after that you should perform the first part of the daily cleansing exercises. These exercises are designed to make you feel the urge to go to the bathroom. These exercises are very gentle, and take 7 - 12 minutes to complete the first set. Then you go to the bathroom and perform the second set of exercises while sitting on the toilet.

The goal of the first set of exercises is to "get the colon in the mood" by loosening up the wastes in the colon. The goal of the second set is to help the large intestine to eliminate its wastes as completely as possible. Both the first and second set of these exercises strengthen the muscles of the large intestine, and activate circulation in all of digestive organs. They are also a very gentle way to wake up in the morning by getting your blood pumping and your mind clear.

You can find the detailed description of the methods of performing these exercises, along with drawings showing exactly how to do each one in my book *Unique Method of Colon Rejuvenation.* The book, *Unique Method of Colon Rejuvenation,* also includes a special diet for the muscles of the intestine. On the following pages are a few sample sections and exercise descriptions from this book, so you can begin right away.

Preparing for the *Cleansing Exercises*

Immediately after rising from bed, refresh yourself by cleansing your mouth and teeth. This should include brushing your teeth, cleansing your tongue and massaging your gums with your fingers (after having washed your hands and fingers carefully).

Next, prepare two big glasses (10 to 12 ounces each) of clean spring water. Set them aside. Then put into a quart-sized glass container two ice cubes made from clean spring water. Now pour the two glasses of water onto the ice in the quart-sized container.

Cut in half one medium-sized lemon. Juice and strain this juice from one half of the lemon. Pour this juice into the water. Stir the water and lemon mixture until the ice melts.

Now pour some of this mixture into one of the two glasses until the glass is almost full. Next pour this lemon water from the one glass into the other glass. Continue to pour the water back and forth in a very thin stream, holding the glasses farther and farther apart, up to about twelve inches apart. This causes the water to absorb vital energy from the air. The water breaks into small droplets which have a greater surface area, permitting the water to absorb more oxygen, which is beneficial to your health and causes it to taste better. Energy from the flowing water converts to energy that will activate and cleanse the digestive system. If possible, do this outside under the rays of the morning sun to enrich the water with even more energy.

Pour the lemon water back and forth three or four times and then drink it. Drink the mixture fairly quickly by taking big sips, but not gulps. With experience, you will be able to finish the first glass in 30 to 60 seconds, but at first just drink as fast as it is comfortable for you. Then, making sure that your breathing is settled, drink the second glass in the same amount of time. Be sure not to drink so fast that you swallow air.

The ice cubes play an important role. First, water from melted ice has special healing power. By mixing it with other water, the energy and information from the ice spreads throughout the mixture. Second, moderately cold water tends to activate the peristaltic action of the digestive system the same way cold pushes us to move and be active in order to create warmth. Upon drinking this water, the coldness in the stomach sends a wave of activity, which spreads through the whole gastrointestinal tract, including the large intestines. It activates the colon's peristaltic action, which is most effective at that time of day.

Keep in mind that whatever is beneficial at one time of day may not be beneficial at a different time of day. For example, deliberately triggering the elimination process later in the day may interfere with digestion. Cold water drunk after a meal tends to hamper digestion since the digestive process needs to reach 102 degrees Fahrenheit to be optimally efficient. This wastes energy since the body must now heat the food back up to temperature. Until this happens, digestion will be "frozen." Strong internal coldness is not helpful to the other internal organs.

The lemon juice also has a very beneficial action in that it alkalinizes and disinfects the digestive system, and is a natural laxative.

Immediately after you finish drinking this lemon-water mixture, begin to do the first part of the Cleansing Exercises. Remember, the main reason for doing these exercises is to create the urge to have a bowel movement.

Bowing to Good Health

1. Kneel so that only your knees and toes touch the floor. (A thin cushion on the floor will protect your knees.) Place your palms on your upper thighs and inhale deeply and slowly. Lower

your body until you are sitting on your heels. Your knees should be a little separated, your body should be upright, and the palms of your hands should be on your knees.

2. While in this position slowly inhale until your lungs are comfortably full. At this point, put your hands against the small of your back. (A man should let his left hand grab his right wrist; a woman should let her right hand grab her left wrist.) Lean over forward, exhaling slowly, arching your back, and touching your abdomen to the top of your thighs. Bend over as far as you can; the ideal is to gently touch your head to the floor.

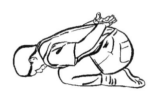

3. Hold your breath in this position for 1 - 2 seconds, or whatever is comfortable.

4. Then rise up slowly while inhaling gently to fill your lungs comfortably. To rise slowly, elevate your head first, then gradually your back, vertebrae by vertebrae. Simultaneously bring your hands from behind you to place them palms-down on your knees.

5. By the end of the inhalation, bring your body back to its original position and relax for the duration of one normal breath.

Repeat this exercise 3-5 times.

Unfolding the Flower

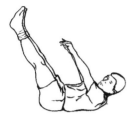

1. Lie on your back on the floor with your legs together and flat on the floor. Put your hands beside your

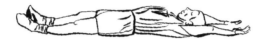

body. Inhale gently but firmly.

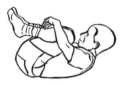

2. As you exhale, bend your knees and bring them toward your head. Embrace them with your arms. (If you are able, try to touch your forehead with your knees.)

3. In this position, inhale through abdominal breathing.

4. Hold your breath for 1-2 seconds.

5. As you exhale, straighten your legs and arms toward a 90° angle to the floor, with the upper part of the body still elevated.

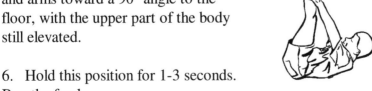

6. Hold this position for 1-3 seconds. Breathe freely.

7. Lower your legs and arms slightly to a 60° angle with the

floor. Hold this position 1-3 seconds.

8. Lower your legs and arms slightly to a 30° angle with the floor. Hold this position 1-3 seconds.

9. Now return to the starting position and relax.

Repeat this exercise 3-5 times. If you have any back problems,

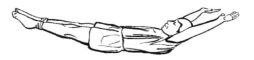

be careful in performing positions #7 and #8.

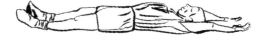

Reaching for the Stars

Part I.

1. Stand upright with your body erect, and with your feet spread about shoulder width apart and pointed forward.

2. With a slow, deep inhalation through the nose, raise your hands above your head. Hold your breath for 1-2 seconds. Make sure you are stretching your torso and arms upward as if you were trying to reach the sky.

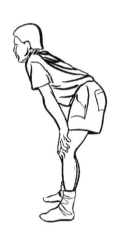

3. While slowly exhaling through your mouth:
   a. Bend your body forward at the waist a little, keeping your back straight;
   b. Bring your arms downward as you bend your body;
   c. Place the palms of your hands on your knees, keeping your arms straight;
   d. Bend your knees a little;
   e. Bring your chin down tightly to your chest.

Part II.

4. Hold your breath for 1-2 seconds and relax your abdominal muscles.
   a. Gravity will tend to pull the abdominal muscles and the organs in your abdomen downward causing them to "drop down."

b. This movement also pulls the diaphragm down, so that automatically and subconsciously you will do a short, silent inhalation through your nose.

5. Right after that, contract your abdominal muscles and push air out through your nose to exhale in short, sharp breaths. (It sounds like you are blowing your nose.)

6. While in this position do a series (10-50) of these short, sharp breaths with full attention to your abdominal muscles. The breaths should be caused by quickly and strongly "bringing in" your abdomen. Relax a couple of seconds and repeat. In the future, you will be able to increase the number of series of this breathing exercise.

Part III.

7. After the last exhalation, do a slow, deep inhalation. At the same time, bring your body to the upright position with your arms raised above your head.

8. With short, forced exhalations through your mouth, bring your arms down. Lips must be almost tight and make resistance to the outgoing air. It looks and sounds as if you want to blow out a candle. Exhale until your lungs are empty.

9. Rest 15-30 seconds and repeat this cycle three times.

Quick Review of Colon Function

The large intestine is basically a long, tubular muscle with the ability to squeeze itself progressively along its length, moving the waste as it squeezes.

Over time, the inside of the colon becomes coated with old, hardened waste, which pushes out the colon walls and resists its muscular contractions. These conditions cause the muscles of the colon to stretch and atrophy.

When a person becomes constipated from old waste accumulated in the colon, he or she may try to overcome this problem by straining. Straining produces improper pressure on the internal organs and may lead to other problems, such as hemorrhoids and anal fissures.

Some people try to solve the problem by taking laxatives. Laxatives irritate the colon walls toward ulcers or more serious problems, and they can create a dependency.

Therefore, in order to improve colon function, the first goal is to remove the source of the difficulty.

To help eliminate as completely as possible, it is useful to do the second set of Cleansing Exercises in the restroom. These exercises will assist and strengthen the weakened muscles of the colon.

Choosing Which Exercise

For most people it is best to perform the exercises as written. However, as you gain familiarity with the different exercises, you will discover which exercises produce the best results in your situation. As you learn the operating principles behind them, you will create variations that are tailored to your body to obtain maximum results for you.

Which exercise is best varies from person to person, and may change for each person from day to day as a result of varying food and other personal conditions. You may notice that material moves through your colon move with greater difficulty in one place than in another. This will be felt as pressure, discomfort or even minor pain. (You can feel this best in a clean, or relatively clean, colon.)

In order to maximize the effectiveness of these exercises, it is helpful to discover where these difficult areas of the colon are for you. The location of such difficult areas will determine which exercises are most appropriate. If, after a few minutes, a particular exercise does not produce the desired results, it is appropriate to go to a different exercise. Remember, never direct pressure in the area of the anus as this can worsen, or even cause, hemorrhoids.

After emptying, the colon muscles relax and rest for a few minutes. In order to help them rest and relax, one of the exercises from the second set, specifically one of those that include arching your back, will be useful.

In order to give your colon extra strength for extra cleansing, it is recommended that you do the following exercises. I have practiced these exercises for years and create new variations all the time. You will find some exercises more productive than others, and will probably use your experiences to develop your own variations. As you practice this second set of exercises you will understand the principles in operation and match these principles to your own situation.

All but the last exercise of the "Throne Room Exercises" involve sitting on the toilet and bending over at the waist. The purpose for this movement is to put pressure on the abdomen using the arms or thighs to stimulate the colon. Generally, pressure is put on the right side first to stimulate movement in the ascending colon. Then pressure is put on the left side to stimulate movement in the descending colon. This follows the natural flow of waste through the large intestine. There are variations of some exercises that call for pressure to be put on the entire colon at one time.

Now, while sitting on the commode in the restroom, begin the exercises of the second set, which are **designed to help you eliminate a large amount of feces without causing tension in the rectal area.** After each exercise, you should rest before going to the next exercise. As a rule, Cleansing Exercises provoke two to four and more ejections from the colon. Always rest after each ejection.

If for some reason you feel that one of these "royal" exercises is not giving you satisfactory results, you will likely need to change your body position. This can be accomplished either by arching your back towards your legs, or by twisting your back to one side or the other.

Try these exercises and see which ones produce the best results for you.

Sample Exercise A

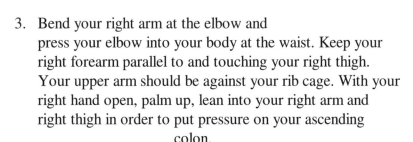

1. Sit on the commode with your body upright.

2. Spread your knees widely but comfortably.

3. Bend your right arm at the elbow and press your elbow into your body at the waist. Keep your right forearm parallel to and touching your right thigh. Your upper arm should be against your rib cage. With your right hand open, palm up, lean into your right arm and right thigh in order to put pressure on your ascending colon.

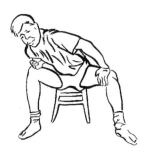

4. Simultaneously, place your left hand on the inside of your left thigh next to your knee. Your left hand should have its palm against your leg, and the fingers on your left hand should be pointing downward. Your left arm should be straight. Push against your left leg.

5. As you are doing this with your arms and legs, arch your back forward in order to put pressure on your ascending colon.

6. Hold this position for 5-10 seconds.

7. Bend your left arm at the elbow and press your elbow into

your body at the waist. Keep your left forearm parallel to and touching your right thigh. Your upper arm should be against your rib cage. With your left hand open, palm up, lean into your left arm and left thigh in order to put pressure on your descending colon.

8. Simultaneously, place your right hand on the inside of your right thigh next to your knee. Your right hand should have its palm against your leg, and the fingers on your right hand should be pointing downwards. Your right arm should be straight.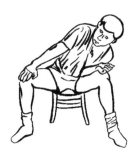

9. As you are doing this with your arms and legs, arch your back toward your legs in order to put pressure on your descending colon.

10. Hold this position for 5-10 seconds.

11. Go back and forth from one side to the other as needed.

Sample Exercise B

1. Sit on the commode with your body upright, legs spread apart.

2. Bend both arms at the elbow in front of you.

3. Make a fist with each hand, using only the fingers and leaving the thumbs extended.

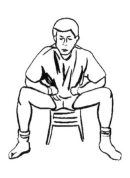

4. Put your fists on the lower part of your abdomen with the thumbs pointing outward.

5. Turn your elbows toward whatever is in front of you so that your abdomen and forearms form a 90° angle (approximately). Make sure the elbows are pointed approximately the same direction as your knees (away from the body).

6. Press with your fists into the lower part of your abdomen.

7. Bend your body forward to put pressure on the entire colon.

8. Try to put your forearms on your thighs.

9. Do slow, deep abdominal breathing, which will increase the pressure on your lower abdomen.

10. Stay in this position as long as you can comfortably, or

until you get results, but not longer than one minute without resting

The Koyfman Twist

Caution: Do this exercise only if you do *not* have a history of back problems. If you do have any kind of back problems, do not do this exercise. When performed, it should be done slowly and carefully, always releasing gently.

1. Sit on the commode with your body upright.

2. Spread your knees.

3. While keeping your left arm straight, place it between your legs, hanging down.

4. Place your left arm inside of the crook of your left knee and grab your left calf with your left hand.

5. Press against the inner part of your left thigh with the back of your left arm.

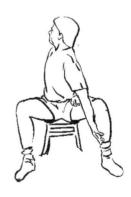

6. Press back with your left thigh against your left arm to increase your ability to twist.

7. Put your right arm behind your back.

8. Bend your right arm at the elbow.

9. With your bent right arm behind your back, carefully try to reach your left hip with the fingers of your right hand.

10. At the same time, slowly and carefully turn the body (right shoulder and head clockwise) as far around as possible. Some people who have more flexibility will possibly be able to reach far enough to grab the inner surface of the left thigh with the right hand.

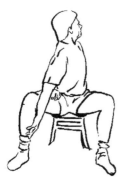

11. Stay in this position a couple of seconds.

12. While in this position, do slow, deep abdominal breathing.

13. Stay in this position as long as it is comfortable. Do not exceed one minute.

14. Very slowly unwind from this position, and rest a few seconds.

15. Perform the same exercise on the other side.

Methods of Colon Stimulation

In order to help the colon to achieve repeated evacuations, the following techniques may be used:

1. Put your hands with spread fingers on your abdomen so that the fingers of one hand are in front of the fingers of the other hand. Press your fingers one by one, creating a wave of pressing and releasing movements on your abdomen. At the same time, try to create some resistance, by bulging your abdomen against your fingers. Breathe freely.

2. Massage your hands in specific places such as the "web" of the hand. This is the fleshy part between the thumb and first finger. Try to massage this area with a circular motion, circling first in one direction and then in the other.

3. **The Lion's Yawn**

   a. Put the palms of your hands on your knees.

   b. Inhale deeply through your nose.

   c. **Slowly** exhale through your mouth. As you exhale, open your mouth as widely as you can, sticking your tongue out as far as you can. This should tightly strain the entire tongue, which is of course a muscle. (This stretch looks like a big yawn).

   d. Hold your breath in this position for a couple of seconds.

   e. Abdominal muscles and arm muscles must be tight.

57

f. Relax and inhale slowly through the nose.

g. Repeat two to four times

    Note: The tongue and the mouth are the beginning of the digestive system. Tension in the tongue, the first link of the system, sends a message throughout the whole chain.

4. Sit up straight and use your hands to feel your abdomen for tense areas. When you find one, press it with your fingers at this specific area with moderate strength. Keep this pressure for little while. If you need to apply a little extra pressure, you can do abdominal breathing at the same time.

Finishing the Evacuating Process

The goal of these Cleansing Exercises is more than to help your colon empty itself. There are other, related benefits as well. These include a feeling of emptiness in the colon that translates into a feeling of lightness in the rest of the body, a sensation of physical comfort that is reflected in emotional well being, and an increase in physical energy due to feeling clean inside.

To make sure that all waste is removed, you need to gently feel your abdomen with your fingers. (Fingers should be perpendicular to the abdomen.) If your abdomen feels relaxed and calm, then your colon is as empty of waste as it can be at the time. It also means you are finished with the morning exercises.

Sometimes colon gases and small amounts of waste remain

in the lower part of the rectum, right in front of the exit (anus). This can create discomfort for the rectal walls and anus. The colon can't create enough pressure to remove this material because there is a very small amount of it.

There is a technique to help your colon to get rid of this remainder and the associated discomfort. Using a small enema syringe introduce 100-200 mg. of clean, purified water into the rectum. Release immediately. This should be done in the standing position. Do not forget to lubricate the tip before introduction.

If the first introduction of the water does not produce the desired results, you may repeat it one or two times. This flushing of the rectal area with a very small amount of water cannot be compared even with an enema. (It is more like rinsing your mouth with water to remove small particles of food after eating.) This simple technique will help maintain your health by helping to prevent hemorrhoids, inflammation of the prostate, etc.

This procedure ends the morning program of cleansing of the large intestine. By learning how to do it correctly and quickly, you will forget what constipation is. You won't want to lose the benefits that this will give you.

Brief Recap of the Morning Program

1. Pour two big glasses with clean, filtered water into a pitcher or other larger glass container.

2. Add to the water the juice of one lemon, and two or three ice cubes made from clean water. (You may want to add the ice earlier so it has time melt).

3. Pour half of this solution into one of the glasses.

4. Pour this half of the solution from one glass to the other, in a thin, long stream. Repeat a couple times, then drink it.

5. Repeat with the second half of the water.

6. Do the first set of Cleansing Exercises.

7. If necessary, go to the restroom and remove the fecal tap from your rectum by using an enema syringe.

8. Do the second set of Cleansing Exercises in the restroom, sitting on the commode. This promotes the emptying of the large intestine.

9. If you feel discomfort, flush your rectum again with a small amount of water using your enema syringe.

Therapeutic Effects of Maintaining the Cleanliness of the Large Intestine

1. Tones the nerves of digestion system.
2. Activates blood flow and strengthens the muscles of the large intestine.
3. Improves the work of liver,
4. Improves the color of your face.
5. Improves your sleep.
6. Freshens your breath.
7. Increases your immunity to diseases.
8. Removes excess gasses.
9. Improves the work of kidneys, lungs, heart and other

organs.

10.   Improves circulation in sex organs.

"Give Him The Nobel Prize"

When I came to the Koyfman center I was desperate and had exhausted doctors and modern medicine for help. I believe that God led me to Dr. Koyfman and his family in Atlanta. I came by car to the center from Denver, CO and stayed for three weeks. When I got there I had serious **sinus and breathing issues.** *I had* **chronic fatigue, depression, digestive problems, unrelenting cravings for junk food, addiction to Nicotine, high blood pressure, terrible pain in my joints and organs that signaled a fake heart attack about 2-3 times a month. I had terrible skin, and could not get off my medications even though I didn't need them, but was chemically dependant. I weighed 290lb** *and because I couldn't sleep and felt so horrible I could not get the energy to get out of bed let alone exercise or do anything recreational. I couldn't get into deep enough sleep to dream, had a bad attitude. I am only 21 yrs of age and could not even make plans for the future more than a day or at the most two.* **After 3 weeks** *of cleansing with the 1ˢᵗ week being no cooperation on my part because I couldn't fast or stop smoking simply due to a lack of will power. But thanks to the Koyfman family's patience and support I fasted and quit smoking the second week, and by the third week I had* **lost 15 lbs,** *didn't crave bad foods, couldn't smoke if I wanted to, slept great for the 1ˢᵗ time in months, had* **no depression, no pain, outstanding energy, breathing fantastically, positive and hopeful attitude and outlook on life. No Medications. Clear thinking, moral clarity and knowledge** *to sustain good health for the rest of my life. I hope that Dr. Koyfman has a blesses and fruitful life and that more people would be trained and dedicated to see others get their health and vitality back with the same selfless attitude and uncomprimising commitment as the Koyfmans. Dr. Koyfman, you and your family and staff are tools in the hand of the Almighty God to change lives and you certainly changed mine. You will see me again and I bless your lives and thank you for helping me and giving me what I need to help many other. Thank you and God be with you.*
Demetrius A. G.
Denver, CO.

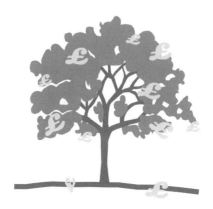

The Kidneys

Things that Lead to Poor Kidney Health

The human body normally has two kidneys. These are located above the waistline in the back of the body on either side of the body. The kidneys are roughly "bean-shaped," and are about the volume of your fist.

The kidneys are important because they filter all of the liquids passing through the body. They remove excess water and toxic substances after the toxins have been neutralized in the liver. Kidneys can remove 6 - 10 cups of liquid. They also regulate pH and mineral levels in the blood.

Things that lead to poor kidney health include not drinking enough pure water to flush the toxins from the kidneys, eating too many foods made from animal products, eating too many processed foods with their artificial chemicals for which the kidneys were not designed, consuming too much protein, etc. Kidney stones develop from these conditions such as these.

Excessive toxins greatly increase the work load of the kidneys, putting them under chemical and physical stress. This stress slows down the normal functioning of the kidney, which results in water retention in the body. Excess water in the body puts extra pressure on the heart, and can increase blood pressure. A weakened heart supplies less energy to the body.

The health of the kidneys depends a lot on the health and condition of the large intestine. Urine channels can be inhibited by pressure from an oversized colon, leading to difficulty in removal of urine. This adds to the retention of liquids in the body.

Ways to Help the Kidneys

It is important to once again point out that our body is one interconnected system. Remember that by taking care of one organ you are also helping other organs.

1. Maintain the cleanliness of your large intestine so that this neighboring organ will not put chemical and physical pressure on your kidneys. (See explanation above.)

2. Prevent blockage in your kidneys by mineral salts and by mucus by drinking sufficient amount of good liquids, especially water, as described above. To determine the average amount of water for an individual to drink each

day, divide the body weight in pounds by 2 and get the amount in liquid ounces that is appropriate to drink. For example: if you weigh 160 lbs., how many glasses of liquids do you need to drink? $160 \div 2 = 80$ ounces; $80 \div 8 = 10$ glasses (because 1 glass = 8 ounces). The proper functioning of the kidneys is also dependent on the level of perspiration via the skin. During the summer the loss of water through the skin is increased so you should drink enough extra water to replace that additional water loss. On the other hand, you can drink a little less water in the wintertime.

How to Spread the Amount of Liquids Throughout the Day

As described above, drink 2 - 3 glasses of water with lemon juice as soon as you awake. Then before lunch and before supper drink 1 - 2 glasses of water 15 - 30 minutes before eating. This can be plain water, water with lemon or apple vinegar, or fresh-squeezed vegetable juice. It is not recommended to drink water during or right after a meal. Water dilutes stomach juice and decreases its capacity to digest food. Because of that you can drink water after a meal only:

30 minutes after fruits,

1½ - 2 hours after starches,

3 - 4 hours after proteins.

During this time it is recommended to drink little portions of water (2-3 sips) every 5-10 minutes so the digestion is not disturbed and the stomach, heart and kidneys are not overburdened. Before going to bed it is recommended to drink 1 glass of herbal tea from chamomile or mint.

What Types of Liquids Can You Drink?

Such popular drinks as coffee, soft drinks, wine, beer and liquor are harmful to your kidneys and to the rest of your body. The best liquid for your body is fresh water, freshly-squeezed fruit and vegetable juices, vegetable broth, herbal teas, extracts from dried fruit and essences from roots and stems.

How to Stimulate Activity of the Kidneys

Massage is a therapy for more than just the muscles. Organ massage done correctly by a trained professional can have very beneficial results for that organ and the rest of the body. Additionally, there are certain basic massage techniques that you can perform on yourself that will also yield benefits. The ones listed below have been practiced for centuries, and will cause no harm unless a person has recently had surgery or has some other extenuating medical situation. In that event, consult your personal health care provider.

The kidneys are one of those organs that can be stimulated in a healthy manner by massage or exercise. To perform this massage on yourself, put both arms behind your back and grab the fingers of one hand with the other hand. With the back of your hands, massage the kidney area using a circular motion until your skin feels warm. The movement can also be up/down or left/right. If desired or necessary, you can massage the kidney area using just one hand or using a massage brush.

Stimulation With Exercises

There are a lot of exercises for stimulating the kidneys. The best ones come from yoga. Below are just three such yoga exercises that have been found to be beneficial to the kidneys.
1. The Cobra.
2. The Grasshopper.
3. The Bow.

In the final position of these exercises, the muscles are tense and blood is pushed out of this area by the pressure from the muscles. When you return to the original position, the muscles relax and blood comes back as a fast moving stream (because tension creates contraction and relaxation releases the "spring"). The stream of blood breaks down blockages and washes out toxins accumulated in that area. Removal of blockages and wastes activates circulation in the area.

The description of these exercises can be found in any book for yoga. It is recommended that you perform at least one of these daily.

What Is Harmful to the Kidneys?

1. Hypothermia, humidity and drafts.
2. Insufficient amount of liquids.
3. Excess amount of liquids.
4. Animal products, meat, cheeses, spicy food, salty fish, canned food.
5. Illegal drugs (and some legal ones).
6. Alcohol in excess.

7. Emotional stress.

What Is Good for Kidneys?

1. Clean water.
2. Hot water with lemon juice.
3. Extract from rosehip.
4. Watermelon juice.
5. Carrot, cucumber and beet juice.
6. Warm baths.
7. Massage.
8. Yoga exercises.

To find out more about kidney cleansing see my book *Eight Steps to Perfect Health.*

What Procedures Are Necessary for Daily Kidney Cleansing?

1. Correctly organized drinking schedule (No, I do not mean alcohol!).
2. Yoga exercises.
3. Some self-massage.
4. Warm shower or warm bath.

Washing not only stimulates the kidneys, but it also facilitates their work by keeping the skin clean. **If the pores of the skin are clean, there will be better perspiration and less stress on kidneys.**

Therapeutic Benefits of Properly Functioning Kidneys

1. Filter toxins from your blood and other tissue fluids.
2. Eliminate salts, excess mucous, uric acid crystals and sand.
3. Increase flexibility in joints and spine.
4. Facilitate work of the heart.
5. Increase sex drive.
6. Increase life span.

"... I have suffered from constipation all of my life. Dr. Koyfman told me that I would need more than just colon cleanses to get rid of my problem, but I was amazed to see that even after my first procedure I felt so much better! I felt light and clean. I was even able to go to the restroom on my own without any laxatives or any other help. His staff is great and very knowledgeable. I can't wait to feel even better..."

Samantha K., 32

"I Passed a Kidney Stone"

I passed a kidney stone (with a lot of pain) while in the hospital. Then I heard about Dr. Koyfman and his natural healing techniques. At that time I weighed 190 lbs (94-95 kg). Dr. Koyfman said that he would try to help me to eliminate another kidney stone, only this time without pain. I didn't believe him in the beginning, but when he explained everything to me, I decided his methods were reasonable and logical. I began the treatment, and passed approximately 150 greenish stones from my liver, mostly size 3.5 cm. I also lost 40 lbs (20 kg). His methods are based on a strict diet, but changing the diet does not mean an absence of food. I knew a lot of massage therapists in Moscow, and Dr. Koyfman is the best.

- Vadim

"Myriad Health Benefits"

Since beginning the cleansing program, I have noticed myriad health benefits: some long standing health problems have lessened in intensity and are on their way to disappearing, while health problems which have developed more recently have disappeared entirely. Dr. Koyfman has never failed in his effort to provide courteous, professional service with a smile that goes "the extra mile." He provides service which gives physical and spiritual benefits. I always enjoy coming here.

- Julie D. Starling

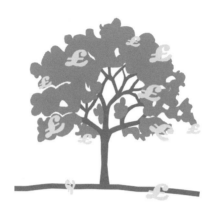

The Lungs

The Role of the Lungs in Nourishment

Healthy human beings can survive without food for one or two months. They can survive five to eleven days without food or water. But no human being can survive more than a few minutes without air. In this context, **breathing in oxygen is the most important nourishment of the body.**

Although we humans do take in air through the skin, the main organ of respiration is the lungs. The human body usually comes packaged with two lungs, one on the left side and one on the right side of the rib cage. The respiratory pathway consists of internal parts of the nose, mouth, trachea and bronchi. The heart, bronchi and major blood vessels are located between the two lungs.

It is very important to breath in through your nose because

while the air is passing through your upper respiratory pathway it gets filtered of dust particles by tiny hair that are covering this pathway. It is also warmed up by being in contact with mucous membranes, rich in blood vessels.

Movement of the lungs is accomplished by the work of the rib cage muscles, and by the diaphragm. The diaphragm is a flat muscle separating the lungs from the abdominal cavity. Just like heart and kidneys, the diaphragm works automatically. But at some level it is possible to consciously regulate the process of respiration.

How Can We Determine the Level of Health by Looking at Respiration?

We can consciously slow down our breathing, speed it up, make it deeper or even stop for some time. The range of this control can be increased with training, cleansing procedures and healthy lifestyle. It is possible to determine how healthy a person is by observing his respiration. **If a person is breathing loudly and frequently when he is at rest, it's a sign of disease. If his breathing is regular, silent and unnoticeable, the person is healthy.** If after exhaling a person can't hold his breath for more than 15 seconds, he is unhealthy. If he can easily hold his breath for 40-60 seconds, then his health is at a good level. If a person can hold his breath for 2-3 minutes and even more, it implies a very high level of health.

How Does the Process of Respiration Happen?

Inhalation occurs when the diaphragm stretches, causing a increase in the volume of the rib cage and lungs. This creates a pressure differential that naturally draws air into the lungs. When the diaphragm returns to its relaxed shape or contracts, the lungs and the rib cage decrease in volume and the air is pushed out. This is exhalation.

How Does the Oxygen Affect Digestion, the Quality of Blood and Cellular Nourishment?

In order to understand this connection we must first examine the process by which blood flows through the body. The heart is the engine by which blood is moved throughout the entire body. This is known as the circulatory system. The blood is pumped through the arteries to the rest of the body down to the cellular level. This is the means by which vitamins, minerals, oxygen, etc. are carried to all parts of the body. The blood then returns to the heart via veins, and from there it is pumped to the lungs where it releases carbon dioxide, and picks up oxygen scavenged from the air we breathe by the action of the lungs.

Oxygen not only nourishes the cells of the body, but also plays a big role in digestion, which heavily depends on oxidizing food once it gets into the blood.

Every particle of food has to be oxidized. Otherwise the body will not get the necessary nourishment, the products of metabolism will not be removed and will poison the body.

So, insufficient amount of oxygen decreases the quality of blood, disrupts cellular metabolism and increases the level of toxicity in the body.

What Is the Quality of Air Which We Breathe?

In centuries past, most human beings spent the majority of their time either outdoors or in houses so well ventilated that it may as well have been outdoors. In developed countries such as the United States, the average person lives in a "canned" environment of processed air. This artificial breathing environment includes a house or apartment whose recirculated air is either cooled or heated, an office under the same conditions, or in a car that heats and cools exhaust-tainted air from surrounding vehicles.

All of these enclosures are heated or cooled by machines which circulate much of the same air over and over again, distributing dust, fibers, pollen and other air-borne contamination. When the air passes through these machines it is damaged by losing some of its natural beneficial characteristics, and picks up some toxic ingredients. But even before it gets to this stage, the air we breathe, particularly in cities, is already polluted by emissions from vehicles of every stripe, aerosols, and numerous biological contaminants such as spores and dust mites. Unavoidably, a great number of offices, hotels and even residential areas are located along major roadways choked with thousands of cars. In addition, factories are adding toxins to our air. In a modern city the cleanest air is found in parks and quite neighborhoods. Despite all of this, the air outside contains more oxygen and more negative ions then the air inside buildings. To make matters worse, the only windows in modern offices that are ever opened are on computer screens, and the amount of time that people spend outside is not much greater than the time it takes to walk from the car to the door of the office or store.

So What Is the Quality of Breathing for the Modern Person?

An inactive lifestyle, such as prolonged sitting at a desk in front of a computer, compresses the rib cage and does not allow the lungs to get a sufficient amount of air. Other things pushing on the lungs and not allowing them to completely open up are (1) an overfilled stomach, (2) an enlarged small intestine and (3) an enlarged colon, as described above. In a person like that, the abdominal organs exert pressure on the diaphragm, which in turn, pushes on the lungs and the breathing becomes shallow and frequent. As a result of this kind of breathing, blood vessels contract, blood circulation is disrupted, limbs become cold.

What Else Disrupts Breathing?

Poor diet produces excess mucous which accumulates not just in the nasal passages but throughout the entire body, and interferes both with respiration and the transmission of oxygen in the body. Unhealthy mucous can be found in the digestive system, kidneys, liver, sinuses, ears, throat, and of course, in the lungs and bronchi. When excess mucous accumulates in bronchi and trachea it makes the respiratory pathway narrower, and air can not move as freely through them as it should. In worse situations, breathing becomes difficult and noisy.

This same **mucous is a prime source of nutrients for bacteria and viruses that invade the body.** If we undergo the negative effects of stress, strong hypothermia or overheating, then these stresses weaken the immune system and diminish our ability to fight infection. That's when bacteria and viruses start to reproduce and spread through our body with a great speed. They feed on mucous, which after passing through their digestive tract, comes out as something different: **toxic mucous.** *Toxic mucous is the reason for many diseases, such as sinus infection; inflammations of the tissues, ears, and gums; diseases of the throat; different inflammatory processes such as flu, fever, and coughing; and a lot of other problems.*

One of the best things we can do to limit the formation of excess mucous is to stop eating mucous-causing foods. These foods include dairy products, pastas, refined grains ,products from refined flour, sweets, fats, and other foods.

How Can You Find Clean Air?

The quality of air depends on its cleanliness and the amount of negative ions available in the air. Most long-lived people (100+ years old) live where clean air is found in abundance. This is usually in the mountains, at the ocean shore or in evergreen forests. Since so much of the population in developed countries lives in the cities, where can one find clean air where millions of cars roam and factories pollute the air?

1. Parks and other areas located far away from busy roads and

air polluting factories are the first choice. Although this air is not ideally clean, it's better than what you will find in buildings or in areas near major roads. Whenever possible (weekends, holidays, etc.) try to get out of the city; and spend some time at less commercialized lakes, rivers, mountains or seashores. There you can take long walks, which are discussed in greater

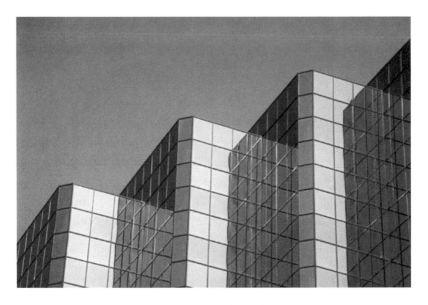

detail below.

2. In your home take whatever steps are necessary to make your air clean. This can include (a) opening windows whenever reasonable, (b) filtering air to remove the toxins that you feel are in the air, (c) installing equipment inside your heating/air conditioning unit to prevent mold and mildew from growing on the moist coils of this equipment and being blown around your home, (d) using pest control products that are environmentally safe and not as toxic to you, (e) checking your

house for molds and mildews that grow behind the walls and have a history of making people sick, and (f) increasing the number of plants in your home since they take in carbon dioxide and give off oxygen. If you sleep in a room where the air is not being refreshed, you may find that you wake up feeling fatigued. This happens because during sleep we exhale carbon dioxide as part of our natural (respiratory) cleansing process. In closed-up rooms, such as most bedrooms are at night, this carbon dioxide can become trapped and concentrated. As we sleep in such an environment, we breathe this respiratory waste back in again. Breathing in too much carbon dioxide has been found to cause people to feel tired, even exhausted, after a full night's sleep. (Remember, carbon dioxide - CO_2 - is not the same as carbon monoxide CO.)

3. In your office, begin working with your organization's management, and the building management, to develop a plan to bring fresh air into the building. Since just leaving the windows or doors open can create very specific problems (decreased security, openings for insects, or increased air toxins in heavily air polluted areas) discussions should center first on the benefits the organization will receive, and then how to bring filtered air into the building. Remind management that poor air makes people tired and therefore less productive. Remind them that sick air makes sick people which translates into more people calling in sick. Remind management that their more talented personnel are just as affected by sick air, so there is no need to encourage them to seek employment elsewhere.

4. The carpet in your house can be the source of molds, dusts, chemicals, irritating fibers, etc. If you can't change the carpets for hard floors, then keeping your carpets clean can become

very important. And yes, this includes frequent vacuuming, and may call for more frequent carpet shampooing. (Be very sure of any chemicals used to clean your carpets.) Frequent carpet maintenance will greatly improve air quality in your home environment.

5. Houses which have basements, cellars or some portion below ground level can become damp, stimulating the growth of mold and mildew. It has been long known that molds and mildews can, and do, make people sick to varying degrees, and it all comes through the air. In such houses it is important to have a dehumidifier or other such machine for pulling excess water vapor out of the air and from the walls. This will go a long way toward helping prevent the growth of mold and mildew.

6. The opposite can also be a problem. If the air in your home, office, etc. is too dry, then it is time to install a humidifier.

7. Check the filters on your air conditioning and heating units. Filters; whether they are kidneys, livers or manmade; are designed to screen out contaminants. That means they are going to get clogged. Therefore, these filters either need to be cleansed or replaced. In the case of filters for air conditioning and heating units, that usually means replacement. Find out what the proper replacement schedule is for your unit, and stick to that schedule. You are worth it.

8. Radon. The word should carry the same emotional impact as the word "Chernobyl." Radon is an odorless, colorless gas given off naturally by certain types of rocks. It results from the decay of radioactive elements in those rocks, and gives off a

radioactive gas. In some areas of the United States, radon levels inside houses has been measured at over 200 picocuries per liter. This is the equivalent of smoking three packs of cigarettes per day! In one area of Tennessee, every other house in one well-to-do neighborhood had family members with lung cancer, and most of these people did not smoke tobacco. Radon gas is impossible for any human to detect by any of the five natural senses. However, there are simple carbon filter devices that can be purchased, or sometimes obtained free from EPA or state environmental agencies that you can use to detect the levels of radon in your home or office. Anything below 4 picocuries per liter is acceptable. Obtain a radon detector today, and follow the instructions exactly. Do not wait for lung cancer to be your first symptom. If you find dangerous levels of radon, seek professional help.

9. Asbestos. Most of the asbestos in the US today has been identified and dealt with. However, a wide variety of older homes and other building are still being found to contain it in the form of insulation for pipes, etc. You (or even better, an asbestos professional) should check for asbestos in your home or place of business. If it is discovered there, you should have a professional deal with it. It is illegal for persons without the proper training and equipment to remove or otherwise handle asbestos. It is an air-borne contaminant whose needle-shaped fibers go into the lungs and do great damage, such as lung cancer. For the average homeowner, it is like finding a dangerous, exotic animal escaped from the zoo inside their home. Don't mess with it. Call for professional help.

10. There are a variety of devices designed to add ozone and negative ions to the air. But no matter how much we try to improve the quality of air, there is no such thing as perfect air

in today's world. The lungs will gradually accumulate toxins, and we need to help our lungs cleanse themselves of toxins.

Methods of Cleansing the Lungs

As detailed earlier, our lungs accumulate a wide variety of harmful substances; such as mucous, manmade fibers, airborne biological contaminants, airborne chemicals, carbon dioxide, second-hand smoke, industrial air pollution, and other things too numerous to mention. As much as we may wish that our lungs would just breathe these toxins back out again, it just doesn't work that way.

The lungs were designed to take in air. Unfortunately, they also take in a whole host of other things with that air because they are exposed to the world almost as much as the skin. Even though they are inside they body, they are not completely shielded from the outside world like the other internal organs. They are exposed to the atmosphere every time we breathe in. Once these toxins are brought into the lungs, many of them don't just stay there. What does not become lodged in the sensitive linings of the lungs is carried by the blood to internal organs, polluting and poisoning them.

However, even if you are breathing the cleanest air possible, there is an additional problem for people living in developed countries. Modern people generally have inactive lifestyles, and their breathing is often very shallow. This is due to internal organs (colon, small intestine, liver, etc.) being overfilled with wastes that crowd the very space of the lungs making less room for the lungs to breathe.

At the same time, the lack of adequate physical exercise, or other significant physical activity, is missing in the lives of most modern persons. Because of this, the lungs are not completely expanded, and stagnant air accumulates in the top portion of the lungs. This has been demonstrated time and time again by cigarette smokers who are able to exhale a small cloud of smoke 10 to 15 minutes after finishing a cigarette merely by consciously exhaling as hard as they can.

This stagnant air and excess mucus in the lungs are ideal conditions for the proliferation of bacteria and viruses. Colds, high fever, cough, flu, pneumonia, and tuberculosis are just some of the problems which result from these conditions. To prevent these diseases it is important to:

1. Maintain the cleanliness of your large intestine and the rest of your digestive system.
2. Eat properly.
3. Use juice therapy and herbs to dilute and eliminate toxic mucus from the lungs and the system.
4. In serious cases, to help the immune system fight infection and eliminate mucus, use a combination of fasting and juice therapy.
5. Maintain cleanliness and freshness of air of your environment.
6. Clean your lungs by deep breathing.

Recipes to Dilute and Eliminate Toxic Mucus

1. Carrot juice (50%), and green juice from celery, romaine lettuce, cucumber, kale, and other greens (50%), plus 1 or 2 cloves of garlic. Drink 3 to 4 cups per day.
2. Black raddish juice. Drink 1 to 3 tablespoons 3 times per day for 1 to 3 weeks.
3. Onion juice (4 oz.), plus organic honey (2 oz.), plus cayenne pepper (1/8 teaspoon). Mix and use 1 to 2 tablespoons 3 or 4 times per day.
4. Horseradish (150 g. (3 oz.) grated), plus the juice from 2 or

3 lemons. Mix and refrigerate; will stay fresh up to 2 weeks. Take ½ teaspoon 2 times per day on an empty stomach. It doesn't irritate the walls of the stomach and does good work.

Technique of Deep Breathing

The simplest way to breathe more deeply is to take long walks in fresh air. The advantages of such walking are: (1) deeper breathing comes automatically and naturally, (2) your heart is not overworked, and (3) your respiration and your heart rate become synchronized. This allows a greater amount of oxygen to be carried by the blood to the cells, supplying them with nutrients.

Techniques of Healthy Walking

1. Clothes. It's important to dress according to the season and the weather. When the temperatures are colder, wearing several lighter layers of clothing is much better than wearing one heavy layer. This is because you can more carefully regulate your body temperature with multiple thin layers than with just one thick layer. As your body warms up from walking, you can remove one or more thin layers to get your temperature just right. Clothing should be made from natural materials, and absorb sweat easily.
2. Shoes. Its best to wear sport shoes and light natural socks. Shoes should be very comfortable and should not hurt your feet.

Times and Places for Walks

As discussed earlier, find a place, such as a park, where air pollution is minimized. Also seek out places that are quieter.

*A unique guidebook published by
Koyfman Whole Body Cleansing*

*Dedicated to your health
and well-being.*

Your health is in your hands

Go Beyond Colonics And The Guidance Of This Book, With Comprehensive Treatment At Koyfman Whole Body Cleansing

This book gives you practical guidance on how to take care of your body, and keep it healthy. If you are looking for comprehensive body cleansing, you may also want to look to Koyfman Whole Body Cleansing in Atlanta for a comprehensive, hands-on approach by experienced specialists.

People come to the Koyfman center from across the country for help with...

- heartburn, indigestion and gas
- constipation
- headaches
- poor nutrient absorption
- constant hunger
- dry skin and itching
- sinus problems and congestion
- seasonal and nutritional allergies
- weight loss
- elimination of parasites: tapeworms, infections, viruses, yeast infections
- cleansing of toxins related to negative emotions
- cleansing from heavy metals
- thyroid imbalance
- general fatigue
- sex drive, prostrate dysfunction
…and more.

Koyfman Whole Body Cleansing has the experience and techniques

to reduce and eliminate these problems from the organs of your body. We go beyond colonics — we treat all organs and systems with unique processes.

At the Koyfman center, we use safe, natural body cleansing methods —

filtered water…proprietary herbal formulas…fresh specialized juices…massage of internal organs…special exercises…FIR "focused organ heating" and infra-red sauna…and specific solutions directed towards individual organs. All these help to dissolve and eliminate the wastes, poisons and blockage in different organs…so your body can remain healthy and take care of itself.

Dr. Yakov Koyfman's unique methods are built on 30 years of experience

The techniques and formulas used at Koyfman Whole Body Cleansing for detoxing the body's vital organs have been developed by Dr. Yakov Koyfman, a naturopathic physician, over a 30 year period of hands-on experience in Ukraine, Russia and Atlanta, Georgia in the United States.

Among his many credentials, Dr. Koyfman has a diploma from the National Board of Naturopathic Examiners, is a European and Oriental Massage Therapist, and is certified by the International Association for Colon HydroTherapy. Plus he has researched methods used by leading natural therapists in India, Russia and Japan, and combines eastern and Western practices.

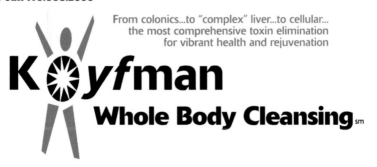

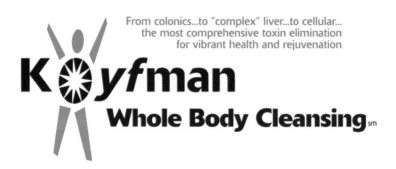

From colonics...to "complex" liver...to cellular...
the most comprehensive toxin elimination
for vibrant health and rejuvenation

K⊙yfman
Whole Body Cleansing sm

*You may also be interested in these other guidebooks from
Koyfman Whole Body Center Publishing:*

Deep Internal Body Cleansing

Healing Through Cleansing 1: Main Cleansing Channels
(colon, kidneys, lungs, skin...)

Healing Through Cleansing 2: Heal and Prevent
(sinus problems, thyroid dysfunction, tooth decay,
ear infection, allergies)

Healing Through Cleansing 3: Healthy Digestion
(stomach, small intestine, liver, blood vessels, lymph...)

Healing Through Cleansing 4: Recipes & Principles
(eating simple, healthy and delicious...)

Unique Method of Colon Rejuvenation

Eight Steps to Perfect Health

*For more information about our books and unique services,
visit us at: www.KoyfmanCenter.com*

Staying away from traffic may be a good mechanism for combining these two. Be mindful of personal safety in all regards.

Air is freshest in the morning as much of the pollution from the previous day's traffic has dissipated. Morning air also contains more energy. After spending the night inside, without breathing fresh air for eight or so hours; morning walks are very important to remove stagnant air, replenish your blood with oxygen and improve your mood. It is also good to take walks in the evening before going to bed.

As the seasons change, the timing for your walks will change as well. In the summertime, it is much better to walk in the morning when it is cooler, than in the heat of the day. Walking when temperatures are very high risks heat stress and heat stroke. Walking during the day, under the blazing sun is not healthy, especially for the skin. Although some sunlight is necessary for good health, too much is a bad idea. Each person is different, so carefully evaluate your own personal circumstances. However, in winter, fall and spring when its not too hot, afternoon walks are a reasonable consideration. Consult your personal health care provider before exercising in extreme temperatures.

How Long Should Your Walk Be?

To start at the basic level, it is better to walk for 5 to10 minutes than to not walk at all. As you gain experience in walking, you should be able to increase this amount of time naturally. By building up to walking for 40 - 60 minutes or even longer you should gain noticeable improvements. Realize that as your body warms up and your lungs begin to breath at the optimal level, even the smallest capillaries open up and greater number of cells receives oxygen.

Walking Technique

While you are walking it is important to keep your body upright and your spine straight. Just imagine that you are hanging from the sky by your head. Your legs should move easily and freely below you while your arms move freely beside your body. Your muscles are relaxed because your mind is concentrating on them being as relaxed as possible. Relaxation helps relieve stress from your muscles, organs and improves the flow of blood. Oxygen and nutrients from food are better carried to every cell.

Breathing Technique During the Walk

If you have the right posture and relax during your walk you will naturally breathe correctly. However, you can consciously help this process by making sure that the air fills up part of abdominal cavity and rib cage. Never try to completely fill up your lungs with air. Excess stretching of lung tissues is harmful. After inhaling hold your breath for 1 - 2 seconds, which is a resting stage for your lungs. After exhaling you can hold your breath for 2 - 4 seconds. During that time the body will use the left over air in the lungs. If you interested in learning more about correct breathing techniques read literature on yoga. But in practice, the kind of breathing that was described here is sufficient for most people.

Technique of Cleansing Respiration

To remove stagnant air from your lungs some people have found it useful to perform cleansing respiration a few times a day. This technique can also be done 2 - 3 times during a walk.

Method

Raise your arms (standing or walking), at the same time slowly inhaling air until your lungs are full. Put your lips together and exhale quickly, as if blowing out a candle. Bring your arms down as you are doing that. Exhale until all of the air is out. Breathe regularly and relax. Repeat the exercise 3-5 times.

One other technique of cleansing respiration is described in the book *Unique Method of Colon Rejuvenation* on page 22 - 23, Exercise 6. This is a multi-orientation exercise, and we will examine its effects in the chapter *"Cleansing of Sinuses and Vessels."*

Meditation During Walking and Jogging

Meditation during walking is a wonderful mixture of movement and relaxation. I have created a meditation program for walking (or jogging) which helps to stimulate meditation. The text of this program is recorded on an audiotape with a pleasant, relaxing, calming music in the background. All you need to use it is a pocket audio player, which would not interfere with movement, and a pair of headphones.

Advantages of the Audiotape Program for Walking/Jogging Meditation

1. You don't have to memorize the program.
2. The text and music have a beneficial effect on the nervous system.
3. The program helps you regulate your breathing, posture, muscle relaxation and energy flow.
4. Because this meditation happens during movement, it activates blood flow and opens up small blood vessels which help satisfy the cells' oxygen needs and cleans them from toxins.
5. This kind of meditation walking is a great way to tone and calm yourself at the same time.
6. The audiotape program teaches a lot of ways for self-hypnosis of positive emotions and cleansing from negative emotions.
7. This meditation will program your mind to protect you in extremely negative situations.

You can order a tape with this program in our office.

Therapeutic Benefits of Clean Lungs

1. Greater immunity to colds and allergies.
2. Improved digestion.
3. Increased oxygen nourishment for cells and organs.
4. Improved blood quality.
5. Reduced amounts of toxins in the body.

6. Heart function strengthened.
7. Normalized blood pressure.
8. Nervous system relaxed and calmed.

"I have had Asthma all my life. It's been slowing me down and restricting in everything I did. Finally, at age 46 I found Dr. Koyfman! This man gave me life. By doing his amazing cleanses and following his dieting recommendations, my symptoms went down to zero in 6 weeks. I am amazed! And the greatest thing about it is that I do not have to rely on cleanses for the rest of my life, all I have to do is keep the asthma free diet that he suggested and use some natural preventative ancient methods. Dr. Koyfman, thank you for your knowledge, for your books and for being here, in Atlanta.
Forever grateful,
Tom Green, 46"

To learn more about unique cleansing procedures done in our center, please visit our website at
www.koyfmancenter.com

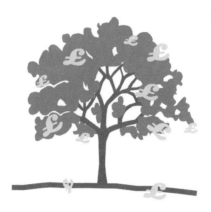

The Skin

What Is the Function of the Skin?

Skin is the largest organ in the human body. And surprisingly enough for most people, the skin is also an excretory organ that helps the body to rid itself of waste.

The human skin has many small openings in its outer surface that are called "pores." It is through these pores that sweat is released to cool the body when it gets too hot. But this sweat also serves another function: waste removal. Toxins in the body are mostly removed by the other excretory organs, but sweat functions as a carrier for toxins in the skin and elsewhere.

In addition, the human skin excretes an oily substance which makes it softer, and maintains its elasticity. (Some people excrete this oil more than others.) As part of the natural growth of your skin, the outermost layer of skin consists of dying cells which gradually fall away and are replaced by new cells. Unfortunately, there are a variety of substances that can become lodged in your pores to block them. For example, dirt and grime from the environment outside of the body, dead skin, wastes from inside the body, natural body oils that have become rancid, fibers from clothing, etc. all can clog your pores and creating favorable conditions for the growth of different kinds of infections.

The excretory function of the skin is intertwined with the excretory function of the kidneys and the lungs. If pores of the skin are blocked and can no longer excrete toxins, then the kidneys have to do extra work, which overloads them and makes them weaker. The same connection exists between the skin and the lungs.

There is also a connection between the health of the skin and the function of the large intestine. If the large intestine is full of wastes, especially long-term wastes, chemicals from the decomposition of these wastes are released into the bloodstream. These unpleasant chemicals travel throughout the body, including to the skin for disposal via the sweat glands in the pores. The chemicals result in an unpleasant smell, especially in the area of feet and armpits. It is for this reason that many people have to use a deodorant to neutralize this odor. **If you cleanse your large intestine, you may find that you won't have to use a deodorant.**

How to Cleanse the Skin

The Dry Approach: Removing dead cells from the skin with a dry brush massage to rejuvenate the skin.

The goal of the dry brush massage is to remove dead skin cells that no longer serve any useful purpose. For that there is a special brush with natural hairs that is your best choice. This massage needs to be performed using light circular movements before taking a shower. The amount of pressure depends on the area of the body you are massaging. You can push a little harder on the back and a little lighter on the stomach because the skin is more sensitive on the stomach, etc. (Do not use the brush to massage your face and the front part of your neck. Women should not massage breasts with this brush. A special massage sponge must be used for the head massage.)

To perform this massage you should brush the arms, back of the neck, head, back (long handled brush), stomach, legs, soles of your feet, and sides of your body. At first use very light pressure, and as your skins gets used to it you can push a little harder. The amount of time needed for this brush self-massage is about 5-10 minutes, or until you feel a pleasant warmth in your skin. After that you can take a warm shower.

A dry brush massage improves the breathing of the skin and makes it smooth and supple.

The Wet Approach: The art of taking a shower.

A warm, gentle shower with a natural soap can also be used as a healthy massage technique to rejuvenate the skin. First get your skin thoroughly wet, and use the shower water to bring your body to the temperature that you find comfortable. Take your wash cloth, get it wet, and put some natural soap on it. Then rub your body lightly with it to apply this natural soap to your body. (To reach your back you can use a brush with a long handle or a special sponge.)

Once you have applied the natural soap to your skin, massage your face, your head and your body with your hands. (Massage your head with the tips of your fingers using circular motions. This will activate blood flow and improve hair growth.) Because your body is covered in soap your hands should easily glide over it. While your hands are employed in this pleasant activity, amplify the value of the massage by forming positive feelings and thoughts from the massage.

Using your hands, lightly massage the bottom of your abdomen, including your sex organs. Organs and glands located in this part of the abdomen are often ignored because too many people fail to separate their clinical (medical) life from their sexual life. A massage in this area is not a sexual activity since that would not relax this part of the body. In fact it would create energy that is not compatible with the purposes of this massage.

Therefore, you should gently massage the bladder, uterus (women), prostate gland and testicles (men), and surrounding areas. Blockages disrupting blood and energy circulation can form in these organs, and a proper massage can improve blood and energy flow to these areas. After you finished with this massage, wash the soap from your body with clean, warm water.

A soap massage in the shower cleans not only the skin but also improves circulation in the whole body and helps its cleansing.

The Hygiene of Massage Brush, Sponge and Towel

Dirt, which you removed from your body, does not always wash down the drain. It can stay on your brush, sponge or towel. If you use those again without cleaning them you will be putting that dirt and bacteria back on your skin. That's why you have to carefully wash and dry them after each shower.

Why Do You Need a Towel in the Bathroom?

Most people in the developed world are trained to dry themselves with a towel as soon as they step out of the shower or bath. Ask yourself if this is a necessity or just a convenience. If you stop and think about it, you would probably say that you just wanted to go ahead and get dry so you could put on clothes and go about your business. But are we missing an opportunity here by so quickly drying off with a towel?

There is another, more effective way of drying yourself. Your hands. First of all, decide that after taking a shower its "ok" not to dry yourself for a little time. Stay wet. This will activate your defense system, and help you become more tolerant of cold. If in a little time after the shower you start feeling cold immediately start to energetically rub your body with the palms of your still clean hands. Then put on your clothes even if there is still some moisture left on your body. You will feel the spreading of pleasant warmth right away.

The Clothes and Health

Clothes which come into contact with your body should be soft, made from natural materials, and be changed daily. They must also be properly laundered.

Clothes made from artificial materials are not able to absorb perspiration nearly as well as natural materials. Since moisture (perspiration) is continuously released by your skin, your clothes need to be able to "wick" moisture away from the body so that your skin can maintain an optimum balance between dryness and humidity. Otherwise the pores of the skin are more easily blocked, and bacteria and fungi will more readily grow on the skin. This can lead to various skin problems and increased body odor.

For the same reason, unnecessary layers of clothing should be avoided since they can trap moisture. In the 1970's, when pantyhose came into vogue, the occurrence of vaginitis increased. This yeast infection was caused by the extra layer of clothing added to the groin area by the panty portion of pantyhose. Alternatives to pantyhose, such as suspender hose and gartered stockings, avoid this particular problem.

Another issue with clothing made from artificial materials is that they become electrolyzed and accumulate static electricity. This electricity can skew the energetic field of the body, resulting in irritability, nervousness and other problems. Clothes from natural materials do not become static and feel nice on your body.

Finally, clothing should never be tight as this merely restricts the flow of blood and other fluids throughout that portion of the body. Traditionally, women's clothes are more notorious than men's clothing in this regard. The elastic bands of brassieres and thigh-high stockings that constrict the flesh over a narrow area are examples of how circulation can be interfered with. Other clothing with elastic bands, and belts that are drawn too tightly, are to be avoided as well. All of these disrupt blood circulation, respiration and digestion.

The Removal of Blockages from Blood Vessels and Different Organs

Why We Get Blockages in the Muscles and Internal Organs

Blockages form in our bodies not only because of incorrect diet, but also from negative emotions and thoughts. Negative emotions and thoughts create a lot of tension in muscles and in internal organs causing a constriction in these areas. As a result the natural flow of blood and other fluids are blocked in small vessels/capillaries, in organ vessels, in internal glands, the bronchi, the digestive system, etc. **Blockages disrupt cell nourishment and cleansing, overload organs, and are the primary reason of many diseases.**

In the digestive system, blockages are caused a variety of factors, such as incorrect food combinations, the accumulation of gases, fatty and carbohydrate products, white flour which turns into a sticky, glue-like mass that clings to colon walls, etc. In the liver, blockages are caused by waste cholesterol and bile, which in time will form bile stones similar to gallstones or kidney stones. In small vessels and glands, blockages can be viscous blood thickened by excessive starches and fats. In bronchi and sinuses it's excess mucous, etc.

To prevent the formation of serious blockages and resulting diseases, it is important to periodically perform deep cleansings of the large intestine, the small intestine, and the liver.

Things You Can Do in Your Bathroom to Break Up Blockages in the Muscles and Internal Organs

Small blockages, which form daily, can be overcome by some relatively simple methods that you can easily do in your own bathroom after a warm shower when your vessels open up from the heat. Instead of drying yourself with the traditional towel, *lightly* tap yourself with your hands to increase circulation. This increased circulation helps to lessen blockages.

The procedure for this "after shower massage" depends on the area of your body you are working. Techniques include using open palms, the knuckles or tips of your fingers brought together and even your fists. (This is NOT self-flagellation, which is not therapeutic.) Light taps relax tense spots and loosen blockages the same way that pulling a cork from a bottle releases pressure. If during your taping of an area (organ) you feel its numbness, continue tapping until you feel it waking up or feel a pleasant warmth. That means that circulation is being restored in that area or organ. To areas where you can't restore sensitivity right away, you have to come back again slightly increasing the force of tapping.

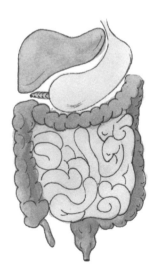

As far as where to begin, start by tapping on your chest in the area of the heart, bronchi and lungs. Then move on to tapping on the liver, gall bladder, stomach, pancreas and spleen. (See graphic for the location of these organs.) Move to the abdominal area (where there is generally a lot of tension), and the area of small intestine at the center of the abdomen. Tapping on the bottom part of the abdomen requires a greater degree of care since this more sensitive area includes the sex organs.

Next, start tapping on your face and forehead. This will help remove blockages from the salivary glands and sinuses. Lightly tap on your head, ears and the back of your neck to remove blockages from vessels in the brain, and in ear canals. This will also activate blood flow in your eyes. Tap yourself on the back, and on your shoulder blades to help your lungs in their cleansing. Then move to your waist and tap your kidneys and adrenal glands. Finally, tap your various joints to help loosen up blockages from uric acid crystals.

Except for the extremely sensitive areas of the body such as the eyes, you will benefit from tapping or massaging every part of the body. In so doing you will pass over energetic centers (chakras) and will also activate their functioning. While you are performing this simple, daily ritual, your mind and your thoughts should be at the same place your hands are. As mentioned earlier, the energy of positive thoughts will increase the effect of the procedure.

This procedure only takes a small amount of time, and is a nice way to bring yourself up to full wakefulness after a morning shower. Most people are surprised to learn that their skin will be completely dry and warm after performing this procedure. The reason for the warmth is the increased circulation of the blood, giving the famous "rosy glow."

Blood Vessel and Nutrients

Vessels are roads by which blood supplies the organs, muscles and cells with nutrients. If these roads are restricted then some of the nutrients will not get to the "consumer" (the cells). These nutrients will settle on the walls of the vessels, and over time decay, until they become toxic. As time passes, the internal condition of such vessels begins to resemble a filled-up large intestine.

This problem sometimes develops from the combination of a poor diet and inadequate exercise, which can cause blood to become viscous (thickened). Thickened blood moves more slowly and can begin to clog-up small vessels such as capillaries. This is a particular problem for those who lead a sedentary life, including the "couch potato," or in computer terms the "mouse potato."

Thickened blood is a concern because most glands are small in size making them too easy to be clogged. The heart has to work harder to overcome these blocks and to pump thickened blood, so it gets tired and weaker faster. Add to this situation the fact that excess table salt is destructive to vessels like corrosion is destructive to metals. This causes vessels to lose elasticity and become fragile resulting in a variety of problems such as increased blood pressure, stroke, heart attack, poor circulation in limbs, spider veins, etc.

It can be said that disrupted blood circulation in organs and cells lies at the heart of any health problem. Depending on one's personal health, one can begin to return to normal blood circulation by first cleanse their large intestine, where a lot of toxins are accumulated, then cleansing their liver and kidneys, which are the primary filters of the blood. This deep internal body cleansing combined with a healthy diet and active lifestyle are the optimum ticket for good health.

Blood Vessel Cleansing in the Shower

It has long been known that hot water applied externally (such as in a shower or bath) causes blood vessels to dilate (or open up). This increases the circulation of blood in the small vessels. Cold water, predictably, has the opposite effect. Cold water causes blood vessels to contract, pushing blood from the small vessels. This expulsion of blood has the effect of removing wastes from vessels.

If one applies hot water followed by cold water in a repeating pattern, one can achieve certain benefits such as making the vessels more elastic and causing more waste to be remove from these vessels. There are other daily procedures for helping to cleanse vessels which we will examine. The important thing to mention before discussing how to correctly perform this procedure is the old saying, "Don't harm your health in pursuit of health."

The best way to implement this particular daily, thermal cleansing technique is as follows:

1. First warm up your body in the shower for one minute in what you fee is warm, pleasant water.
2. Follow this with cooler water for 15 to 30 seconds.
3. Then increase the shower water temperature to "pleasantly hot" for one minute, and lower it to "pleasantly cool" for 15 to 30 seconds.
4. This cycle of pleasantly hot-and-cold-water should be repeated five to seven times, and more if you feel so inclined.
5. Finish your shower with cold water.

It is important to keep in mind that the water temperature should not be too cold or too hot. Avoid extremes. It is also important to learn to change the temperature of the water quickly without burning or freezing yourself.

By using this procedure correctly you can expand the good effects of heating and cooling on your body. This will strengthen your body and will make it less susceptible to disease. This procedure cleanses blood vessels, cleanses the skin, and fills your body with energy.

But if you go to extremes by excessively lowering the temperature you will end up with a cold, nasal and sinusoidal congestion, etc. On the other hand if you make the water too hot you can overheat or even burn yourself. So, you should follow the same basic principle when performing any procedure, exercise, diet, etc. Be moderate. Follow your feelings and common sense, and you will achieve optimum health.

Therapeutic Effects of Clean Skin

1. Makes kidneys' work easier.
2. Makes lungs' work easier.
3. Skin becomes soft and nice smelling.

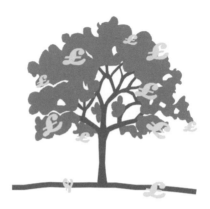

Moderation

Moderation Is a Form of Balance

Too many people throughout the world believe that the bigger, the faster, the further, the stronger, etc, something is, the better it is. This can sometimes be applied to "things," but it can not be safely applied to the human body. The classic example of this is the typically short life span of Olympic athletes. To "get the gold," these incredible athletes too often burn up their lives by pushing their bodies to the extreme limits.

Of course, expanding the borders of human abilities is very important. Without the courageous daring and heroic efforts of many pioneers throughout the millennia, we would still be in caves both physically and otherwise. The question is how and where to balance everything in order to get the most out of life.

Moderation is the key in terms of human health and longevity. Going beyond the limits is great for setting records, but harmful to personal health. Even getting close to one's limits is dangerous because it uses up the body's reserves of stored energy. Those reserves are there for emergencies, and tapping them is like spending your money down to the last dollar. If those reserves are used too frequently or too deeply, the stored energy is depleted, and the door is opened to becoming sick in so many ways. For most people this means that you made yourself sick while trying to make your body stronger, healthier, cleaner, etc. and you harmed your health.

Athletes

Again, the best example of this is athletes who seem to thrive on pushing themselves to the limit, and seeing how far they (their reserves) can go. This is often done for pride and perceived "glory." There are also those people who are so competitive that they have to compete with somebody or something, even if it is just competing with themselves or with numbers. While those around them think that athletes are strong and healthy, if you follow their lives you will see that they often have heart disease, joint injuries and pain, migraines, etc. Life span is often shorter for athletes than for those who are not involved in sports. But is it worth it when you see how they really "finish?"

The question then becomes, "How do I know when to stop?" The answer is simple, "Follow your feelings." If your activity gives you a "high," but you still don't feel very good, then you lost. On the other hand if your activity did not give you the exercise "high" or you didn't do as well as before, but you feel great, you won.

Ask yourself this question, "What are my real goals?" If
your goal is to get some super body shape for so short a time as
a few years just to impress someone else (including strangers)
and it is at the expense of your long term health, is it worth it?
Is it worth having the second half of your life filled with pain
when you walk, etc.?

Real Competition

If you really want to compete, compete with something
grand, like life itself. Don't waste your time competing with
mere numbers such as, "Can I run this distance a minute
faster," or "Can I lift five more pounds," etc. Compete for
quality of life in the form of a pain-free life with no joint pain
or torn ligaments or damaged muscles. Compete for quality of
life in the form of an internally clean body that has a
powerhouse immune system that can run circles around colds
and other sicknesses so you can enjoy more days. Compete for
a quality of life that gives real dignity to growing old in years
(aging like wine) instead of growing old in physical disabilities
because you ate junk food that poisoned your body (aging like
cheese). Compete for a balanced life based on moderation in
diet, exercise, and internal cleanliness that gives you a long
span of life.

You only get one life, and you want to have the best
physical health you possibly can so that every other aspect of
your life is amplified. You are the only one who can make
these decisions. You are the only one who can save your life.
There is no need to "sell out" to bad lifestyle practices just to
please your taste buds, or go along with the crowd, or to feel
like Superman/Superwoman to impress your ego. Get the

happiness now that comes from real satisfaction; that comes with balance not extremes. Life is a journey, more than a goal. Make these two into one so that the good journey you are making is the goal itself. So if someone can lift more than you, run faster, etc, don't feel inadequate. They aren't the reference standard for your life anyway. The maximum you can achieve without damaging your self is a much better reference standard than other people or the measurements of time, weight, speed, etc. Focus instead on the measurements of health, energy, clear mind, light fresh breath, feeling young, great mood, etc.

The Next Book

In many ways our health depends on the health of organs located in the head and neck regions: the brain, thyroid gland, eyes, salivary glands, ears, nose and sinuses, throat, tongue, teeth and gums. Our health also depends on proper connection between the brain and other internal organs.

The contemporary American diet usually includes a large number of mucus-forming foods that result in the generation of mucus through-out the body. Excess mucus settles throughout the body, especially in the head and neck organs giving rise to a number of ailments in these organs. Negative thoughts and emotions can destroy the connection between the brain and other organs and lead to various diseases.

How can you help your organs located in your head and neck regions to become free of toxins and sustain the health of your entire body? You will find the answers in the pages of *Healing through Cleansing, Book 2*.

Other valuable information in this book includes:

• How to Restore Proper Connection Between the Brain and

Other Parts of the Body for Better Functioning.
- How to Improve the Function of the Thyroid Gland, the Main Fortress of Your System.
- Simple Way to Cleanse Your Blood Every Day.
- How to Prevent Tooth Decay and Prevent and Heal Bleeding Gums and Gingivitis.
- Simple Way of Helping with Pollen Allergy.
- And Much More . . .

"...passing that kidney stone was not exactly fun, but I am glad I did it without surgery or other strange medical procedures and medications. Dr. Koyfman's technique is very gentle and doable for anyone. Even before I got to the actual kidney cleansing, doing all the preparation cleanses made me feel much better. I did not have so much discomfort and pain in my kidneys. My sex life had improved drastically. I had more energy, etc. During my actual kidney cleansing, I started passing sand and small stones. Because of the good preparation the stones were mostly dissolved and broken down into small particles, which helped me pass them much easier. I am so glad I chose this method. I am a new man!"

Bob C.

Testimonials

"Bronchitis for Over Ten Years"

I have suffered from bronchitis and respiratory problems for over ten years. I was sick with bronchial infections for several weeks at least twice every year. Medical doctors repeatedly told me that I had chronic bronchitis, and they treated the condition with antibiotics. However, my immune system became weakened, and I was constantly sick with colds and laryngitis. It appeared as though the antibiotics had become somewhat ineffective. As the bronchial condition worsened, I was diagnosed as having asthma.

After suffering from asthma for almost a year with my doctor treating the disease with steroid pills and several types of nasal and oral inhalers, my condition had grown progressively worse. I became weakened from coughing, wheezing, and choking for air. I would awaken from my sleep coughing and choking during the night. I could hardly climb a flight of stairs without becoming short of breath, weak, and tired. I felt helpless and honestly thought that I was going to die from this disease.

It was absolutely a providence that my daughter worked for a naturopathic doctor during this time. My daughter advised me to see this doctor. Although I was not quite familiar with natural healing then, I knew that I desperately needed help and went to see the doctor. After consulting with me the doctor said, "You are full of toxins. Your eyes are puffed. Your face is swollen. Your joints are stiff and swollen. And you are bloated. You need to see Dr. Koyfman." The doctor's nurse called Dr. Koyfman's office and made an appointment for me. I saw him that very afternoon.

The year was 1999. It was the week before Christmas when Dr. Koyfman began treating me. After just a few treatments of colonics I began to breathe better and feel stronger. Dr. Koyfman developed a treatment plan to fit my need and care, and I began the program with focus and discipline. Now almost a year later, I am honored to testify to the world and say that I no longer take medications for asthma and palpitations. My blood pressure and cholesterol results are normal. I have lost 30 pounds. I am lean, stronger, and full of energy, but most of all I am well and healthy.

Dr. Koyfman is an excellent Naturopathic Doctor and teacher. In my opinion, he is one of the best doctors in his business. His ultimate objective is to restore patients' wellness. Dr. Koyfman taught me how to take better care of myself. For example, I learned the value of exercise, how to adjust to a healthy lifestyle, and most of all the wholeness of food.

Dr. Koyfman and his staff care about their patients and provide their patients with excellent service. I am grateful to Dr. Koyfman for my wellness and my quality of life. I feel that God has healed me through Dr. Koyfman's hands. I am thankful to Mrs. Koyfman for her support and excellent care, and to Alex for his kindness and good cheer during the difficult times.

—Joyce Martin
November, 2000

"Within Three Days, Wheezing Gone"

I have been a client of Dr. Koyfman's for one short month, and during that time I have had great success with his natural healing methods, diet, exercise, and internal body cleansing.

I was skeptical, but was ready to try anything since I was having no luck with traditional medicine.

I had a chronic cough, wheezing and shortness of breath for one and one-half years. I had been to five separate specialist over that time and was diagnosed with allergies, asthma, and acid reflux. I tried medications for each problem with no results. The coughing/wheezing would not go away.

I was very frustrated and felt that the doctors would not listen to me. I knew that this was not acid reflux, but they insisted that it was even though several tests showed no reflux. I knew in my heart that I had to find a better way to heal myself, and Dr. Koyfman became the answer to this complex equation.

My chiropractor referred me to Dr. Koyfman, and that referral changed my life. I stopped taking supplements from my chiropractor and started a healing diet. I had my first colonic and within three days the coughing/wheezing was completely gone. Because of this, my life has hanged for the positive. I feel as though I have been reborn. I have so much more energy and a much healthier outlook on life. I still have a lot of work to do, but I now have hope that I can live the next half of my life healthy and disease free. Thank you, Dr. Koyfman.

—Donna Creel, 41
Woodstock, GA

"Grandson, Grandmother, Entire Family"

Our grandson was having great difficulty breathing, and was supposed to have sinus surgery. Instead, we brought him to Dr. Koyfman who worked with him for a little over two months. Now our grandson is breathing normally and is healthy. Dr. Koyfman's natural techniques helped us avoid the expense, trauma and scarring of surgery. I (the grandmother) went through the liver cleansing procedure and was astonished to see the green stones that came out of my body. This helped me to understand what was really going on in my body and to understand the benefits of Dr. Koyfman's treatments. I also lost 40 pounds (20 kg). Dr. Koyfman is the perfect massage therapist, and is a qualified specialist in his area. He has a quick mind He works with everyone individually, and gives a lot of good suggestions. Now the entire family has changed our diet to healthier foods. Yakov is a Godsend.

—Family M., Family of Five
All of Whom Participated in Our Services

"With Just the Touch of His Hands"

I had done a lot of reading about natural healing before I ever got beyond the stage of just nutritional supplements. I knew that my body (just like everyone else's) had the nasty habit of storing wastes in the colon, liver, kidneys, and other organs down to the cellular level. I knew I had to find a way to flush these wastes out by natural means (like colonics) but who had the training, skills and experience?
Then a friend recommended Dr. Koyfman to me as someone with exceptional skills in colon hydrotherapy. She had been to

other colon hydrotherapists, and had had bad experiences. So I took the plunge and made an appointment for my first colonic. I was pleased to see that everything was done hygienically, and that there was no pain involved. I was also pleased that there were no odors or mess. I was amazed during the procedure that Dr. Koyfman had what most people would refer to as "the touch." With just the touch of his hands he could feel my abdomen and tell where the wastes were. Then he would massage that area to loosen it up. The results were "productive."

But what I really liked was seeing the old, black wastes that had been stuck to my colon wall for years and years go floating through the colonic machine and down the drain forever. After I had finished the basic series of colonics I ended up losing a minimum of 15 pounds of dangerous, toxic wastes that had clung to my colon wall, and another ten pounds of regular (fatty) weight as well.

After that I did the small intestine cleanse, the liver cleanse and the kidney cleanse. I admitted to Dr. Koyfman that I was a skeptic about the liver cleanse, but the visibly obvious effectiveness of the liver cleanse eliminated all doubts. All of the four liver cleanses flushed out small (about the size of a new pencil eraser) stones that were either black or green. The black stones were football-shaped and they predominated during the first three liver cleanses. But during the fourth liver cleanse, the green stones really started to come out. Hundreds of these black stones have been flushed out during the first three cleanses, but the fourth cleanse flushed out at least 100 by itself. Also, about a quarter cup of sand-sized liver stones were flushed out.

The idea that my body does not have to fight these toxins 24-hours-a-day, seven-days-a-week gives me a great sense of well-being. No longer are these wastes releasing toxins into my bloodstream and overwhelming my liver with unnecessary work. Now my body can get about the more important business of protecting itself from everyday, new toxins that come into the body unbidden all of the time. I feel better, have lost weight, my sinuses have improved dramatically, and people tell me I look younger. On top of that, I believe my chances of getting cancer are greatly reduced. This is perhaps the best investment I could have made; in my own health.

- Jack, Professional Scientist

"Dealing with the Stress of My Lifestyle"

I have been a client of Dr. Koyfman's since 1996 and during that time I have been impressed by the fact that he is the most professional and courteous doctor that I have ever dealt with. He has helped me immensely with his "Deep Internal Body Cleansing" techniques and procedures.

Before I went to Dr. Koyfman I was having a rough time dealing with the stress of my lifestyle and the stress of my business. As difficult as it might be to believe, if it were not for Dr. Koyfman's liver cleansing procedures I believe I would have either killed someone or tried to kill someone.

Because of Dr. Koyfman's non-invasive detoxification program, I am better able to function as a normal person and get along in today's society. Dr. Koyfman is an asset to the community. His techniques and knowledge can only help others like myself that are forced to deal with the constant tensions and toxins that come along with living in today's world.

Note: Vinny had a record in our center by fasting for 85 days. Five years later, another lady overpowered him by fasting 140 days.

Vinny Conzo. 1986 winner of the "Mr. U.S.A." title.

Before coming to the Koyfman Center, I was very constipated. My bowel movements were only 1-2 times per week. After my program at the Koyfman Center, I now have 2-3 bowel movements per day. My energy level is better than it had been in 10 years. I am vary pleases with my results. The staff is very nice and knowledgeable of the services offered. Thanks everyone for an enjoyable experience that I will never forget.

-- Kay M –
Tampa, Florida

Since I started coming to the Koyfman Whole Body Cleansing for my procedures and was guided to a proper diet, all my problems just disappeared. It was amazing. Only a few visits and my hot flashes were gone for good, liver sourness was gone, I've lost 35 pounds in about 2 months and my energy jumped through the roof. I feel better and younger than I ever did in my life.

Luda. Age 56 Chicago, IL

"My Colon Was Unable to Function"

I am a 44-year-old wife and mother of two. We recently experienced a fire in our home which put my 75-year-old mother (who suffers from emphysema) into the hospital where she was put on a life support system for a week. My mother survived this, and the rest of us escaped unhurt. However, the stress and trauma of this experience sent my body into shock and my colon was unable to function. At first, I wasn't too concerned, and after a couple of weeks I was very worried. Needless to say, I was giving myself a daily enema. When I went to Dr. Koyfman and told him of my situation, he calmly told I would be fine if I did a series of exercises described in his book to strengthen my colon. I did the exercises and was perfectly fine in about ten days and feel stronger and healthier than ever. I also followed his other recommendations and techniques described in his Healing Through Cleansing Book series.

I am amazed that just by doing simple things at home on my own at my own convenience.   -Donna .M., California

"I Had a Water Retention Problem"

Energized! I had a water retention problem and with my first treatment I noticed an enormous amount of excess fluid. I saw a noticeable decrease in weight. I had first delivered a baby three weeks prior. People have noticed the difference. I would recommend this procedure to anyone who is looking for an alternative to traditional medicine for a variety of maladies. I will continue with my treatments. They definitely have given me energy and more resistance to daily stress.

Katherine Phelps

Publisher, Today's Atlanta Woman

"Pacemaker at age 60"

Doctors have only one answer to all questions–surgery. I had some problems with my heart, but refused the surgery and didn't feel like having something hooked to my heart. I was very overweight and bloated. My energy was low and doing anything felt like a drag. After having a conversation with Dr. Koyfman, I felt confident in his knowledge and ability to help me. After only a few visits, I was a new man. I've lost more weight than I ever hoped for. My water retention is gone. I do not have any heart problems. I can ride my bicycle again and even uphill is not a challenge anymore. Anyone who sees me can't believe that within two months I lost 20 years. I am energized, healthy and young again.   Don B. Age 62

Unique Method of Colon Rejuvenation, 95
pages; $12.

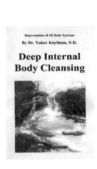

Our bodies need constant help eliminating
toxic substances which enter the system every
day. Daily practice of the rising and restroom
exercises described in this book strengthens
colon muscles so that, with time, elimination
will accompany each meal and eject more toxins
than are retained. Also included are principles
and recipes for healthy eating, raw meals, and safe cooking
technology.

**Eight Steps to Total Body Cleansing and
Perfect Health,** 214 pages; $20.

You will find here how to prepare for
cleansing and what to expect during Deep
Internal Body Cleansing. You will want to know
what to do if you feel any discomfort during the
cleansing. This book explains how we perform
Deep Internal Body Cleansing at the Center.
Also, you will discover here what to eat after the
cleansing in order to maintain your success and your new
lifestyle.

Deep Internal Body Cleansing, 172 pages.
$15 plus shipping and handling.

If you search for healing and real health, then
here you will find answers to your questions
Here is information about toxicity and the
immune system, healthy eating and eliminating
parasites. Here are answers to help you resist
hurtful cravings and negative emotions. You
really can get health and gain energy through
cleansing your body.

Healing Through Cleansing - Book 2, 101 pages; $12.

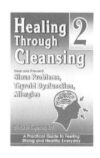

In many ways our health depends on the health of organs located in the head and neck regions: the brain, thyroid gland, eyes, salivary glands, ears, nose and sinuses, throat, tongue, teeth and gums. The contemporary American diet usually includes a large number of mucus-forming foods that result in the generation of mucus throughout the body. Excess mucus settles throughout the body, especially in the head and neck organs, giving rise to a number of ailments in these organs.

Healing Through Cleansing - Book 3, 120 pages; $12.

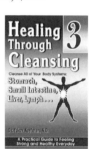

The abdominal area is the kitchen of our bodies. How well or poorly this kitchen functions depends on whether we feed our system with nutrients or poison our system with toxicity. If your abdominal kitchen produces nutrients, you are getting health; if your kitchen produces poison, you are getting disease. How can you help your abdominal organs to become more healthy and free of toxins and to sustain the health of your entire body? You will find the answers in the pages of this book.

Healing Through Cleansing Diet - Book 4, 116 pages; $12.

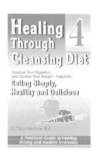

"To get the best results in the healing process, it is not enough to find a skilled teacher who can guide you along the path. It is also very important that the student be open-minded to new information and ready to work," says Dr. Yakov Koyfman, N.D. A healthy diet gives to the system not only nutrients but also help to clean and heal the body. To make your diet healthy, you need to learn the things in this book.